Knowledge for contemporary nursing practice

For Mosby:

Senior Commissioning Editor: Sarena Wolfaard
Project Development Manager: Mairi McCubbin
Project Manager: Ailsa Laing
Designer: Judith Wright
Illustrations Manager: Bruce Hogarth

Knowledge for contemporary nursing practice

Patricia Cronin MSc BSc(Hons) DipN RN
Senior Lecturer, St Bartholomew's School of Nursing and Midwifery, City University,
London, UK

Karen Rawlings-Anderson MSc BA(Hons) DipNEd RN
Senior Lecturer, St Bartholomew's School of Nursing and Midwifery, City University,
London, UK

Foreword by
Professor Hugh McKenna PhD RMN RGN DipN(Lond)
AdvDipEd RNT
Head of School, School of Nursing, University of Ulster, Newtownabbey, UK

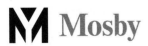 Mosby

EDINBURGH LONDON NEW YORK OXFORD PHILADELPHIA ST LOUIS SYDNEY TORONTO 2004

MOSBY
An affiliate of Elsevier Science Limited

First published 2004

ISBN 0 7234 3275 9

British Library Cataloguing in Publication Data
A catalogue record for this book is available from the British Library

Library of Congress Cataloging in Publication Data
A catalog record for this book is available from the Library of Congress

Notice
Medical knowledge is constantly changing. Standard safety precautions must be followed, but as new research and clinical experience broaden our knowledge, changes in treatment and drug therapy may become necessary or appropriate. Readers are advised to check the most current product information provided by the manufacturer of each drug to be administered to verify the recommended dose, the method and duration of administration, and contraindications. It is the responsibility of the practitioner, relying on experience and knowledge of the patient, to determine dosages and the best treatment for each individual patient. Neither the Publisher nor the authors assume any liability for any injury and/or damage to persons or property arising from this publication.

The Publisher

Printed in China

 your source for books,
journals and multimedia
in the health sciences

www.elsevierhealth.com

The
Publisher's
policy is to use
**paper manufactured
from sustainable forests**

Contents

Foreword

It is a great honour to be asked to write the foreword for this important book. It is a truism that in the future nursing will not be taught or practised the way it has been hitherto. In 1952 Virginia Henderson set out to collect all the research papers written in nursing. When her task was complete she had only managed to fill two slim volumes. Fifty years later, I suspect that it would take two large buildings to house all the nursing research published in the interim. This signifies the exponential growth in the development of the knowledge base for nursing practice.

Nursing is an applied discipline and knowledge is of little use if it has no implication for or impact on practice. Our continued existence as a profession is based entirely on how we can improve the health and well-being of patients, their families and their communities. Therefore, the link between our knowledge base and our practice stands at the core of our survival as a discipline.

For some time now, I have been aware of the work of Patricia Cronin and Karen Rawlings-Anderson. They are very experienced scholars and have produced a user-friendly book that weaves the nature of knowledge with the nature of practice. Almost like a double helix, knowledge is linked to practice in an interdependent way, so that as knowledge changes so also should practice. This cause and effect relationship between knowledge and practice is a two-way process and this message permeates the text. What is particularly interesting is that this relationship is set within the wider socio-political culture of modern health care, where issues such as the changing workforce, clinical governance, codes of practice and organisation of care are influencing nursing's work.

I suspect that the stimulus for this book has been the excellent feedback that the authors have received from students. However, there is always a risk that good teaching materials do not transfer well into a good textbook. In *Knowledge for Contemporary Nursing Practice,* nothing has been lost in the transition. The book is expertly crafted and its easy style and 'readability' are some of its most pleasing features. The activity boxes and key points give structure to the book, as well as helping to engage its readers. Its slim volume will be acceptable to many health professionals who are turned off by the normal heavy US tomes on the subject. The short chapters are interesting and authoritative and can be read on a 'stand-alone' basis, allowing readers to 'dip in and out'.

This book has arrived at an opportune time. Nurses are being encouraged to underpin their clinical decision-making with best evidence. Furthermore, clinical governance has ensured that out-of-date knowledge has no place in modern health care. To practice without being aware of the most up-to-date knowledge would be like starting a new journey without a map. This book is one of the best maps of the knowledge–practice terrain that I have come across. I congratulate Patricia and Karen on producing it.

Professor Hugh McKenna
Head of School of Nursing
University of Ulster 2004

Preface

The overall aim of this book is to facilitate the exploration and understanding of theoretical and professional issues that have relevance for contemporary nursing practice. As teachers of nursing, we have come to recognise that many nurses believe that, although they need to know about nursing theory and professional issues in order to complete nursing courses, they have little relevance for everyday practice. It is our contention, however, that the practice of nursing is not an isolated endeavour, but happens in a socio-political world whose influences are pervasive. A failure to understand or locate nursing in this context leads nurses to have difficulty in articulating what it is they do and what their unique contribution to health care is. Moreover, with the move towards competency-based education, there is a danger that the theoretical underpinnings of nursing will be lost.

Currently, this area of the market is dominated by texts from the USA. While being theoretically useful, many students find the language difficult to understand and the care context inappropriate to health care in the UK. Several UK texts focus on nursing theories and models or professional issues, but none encompasses the relationship between the two areas. We hope that this book will go some way towards demonstrating the relevance of both theory and professional issues to the reality of practice. Unlike texts that merely present these issues theoretically, this book will focus on both their meaning and application to practice.

The book is divided into two sections: the first deals with the nature of nursing knowledge, and the second focuses on the nature of professional nursing practice. The relationship between the two sections is signposted by cross-referencing within chapters. Examples from nursing practice are used to illustrate the relevance of the issues being discussed, while activities for the reader are included to enhance understanding.

Nursing, since the mid-twentieth century has been very concerned with knowledge and what knowledge is important for the discipline. Chapter 1 gives a brief history of philosophy, considers the four main areas of philosophic inquiry and locates the debates about nursing knowledge. Significant influences on nursing and its development are discussed, and some insight into why we are where we are today is offered.

Chapter 2 continues this exploration by articulating some of the debates regarding knowledge in nursing. An overview of 'what is knowledge?' or 'what counts as knowledge?' is presented, the complexity of which becomes evident. The view that the western traditional view of knowledge, 'knowledge that' or propositional knowledge does not account for all the knowledge needed by the nurse in clinical practice is explored, and key texts by Belenky et al (1986), Benner (1984) and Carper (1978) are presented.

Chapter 3 focuses on theory in nursing with the contention that theory provides knowledge about the world and provides a structure for the generation of knowledge that is important to a discipline, as well as providing direction and organisation. The purpose of the chapter is to attempt to unravel the world of theory beginning with an exploration of 'what is theory?' and an examination of 'what is nursing theory?'

Chapter 4 examines the relationship between theory, research and practice with a particular focus on the theory–research links. The interdependency between the three concepts is explored and includes a brief insight into the nature of research. In a practice-based discipline such as nursing, it is proposed that theory provides knowledge about the world of clinical practice through research. Strategies for theory generation and theory validation are presented in order to structure the links.

Chapter 5 is concerned with the importance of attaining conceptual clarity in nursing practice. The value of concept analysis is outlined and two frameworks for concept analysis are presented. The use of published concept analyses to enhance individual practice is examined through a series of activities related to the concept of hope. The chapter concludes with some self-directed activities for the reader.

In the second section, professional issues that are of concern to nurses are explored. Chapter 6 discusses the nature of professional nursing practice within the context of the changing health-care arena. The debate relating to whether nursing is a profession is examined and related to the contemporary role of the nurse. The issues of responsibility; authority; autonomy; accountability and expanding roles are discussed in relation to the Code of Professional Conduct.

Chapter 7 considers how nurses make decisions in their everyday practice. The nursing process as a problem-solving approach to nursing is reviewed and critiqued, and the move towards using integrated care pathways is explored. The range of skills required to make effective clinical decisions is also examined in relation to the level of expertise and experience of the nurse.

Chapter 8 moves on to look at how care is managed. Individual nurses may prioritise their own workload, but care must be managed in such a way as to ensure coordination of services and continuity for the patient. The chapter explores task and patient allocation, team nursing, primary nursing and case management. The development of new roles for nurses aimed at improving the management and delivery of care are also explored. In light of recent government initiatives, the wider context of organisation of care is reviewed and clinical governance is discussed.

Chapter 9 explores the notion of reflective practice, and how we use our existing knowledge and experience in clinical situations. The chapter investigates what reflective practice entails, and considers its merits and shortcomings. Frameworks that may facilitate the reflective process are used in exemplars of reflective writing, and the links between reflective practice and critical thinking are examined.

To summarise, the purpose of this book is to elucidate the many theoretical and professional issues that influence our everyday practice. The book is born out of our belief that nursing has the potential to offer a unique and distinct contribution to health care. We have resisted the temptation to preach in a dogmatic manner, but have instead attempted to offer a book that can be used by both pre- and post-registration nurses to shed some light on issues that are often complex. This book can be referred to and revisited as the reader's interest and need for deeper understanding of the influences on their practice develops.

Patricia Cronin
Karen Rawlings-Anderson
London 2004

Acknowledgement

We would like to thank our colleague Anne Manning for her support during the writing of this book. Her advice and critical reading skills were invaluable.

The nature of nursing knowledge

Section 1 begins with a brief exploration of the history of philosophy and is followed by a consideration of the nature of nursing knowledge, theory in nursing and its relationship with research and practice. The section concludes with an examination of concepts and concept analysis.

SECTION CONTENTS

1

Why is philosophy relevant to nursing?

INTRODUCTION

This section of the book is concerned with the nature of nursing knowledge and its structure. When you chose to become a nurse, you will have had some conception of what a nurse is, what nurses do and perhaps what you would be learning. At times you may question the relevance of what you are expected to learn. For example, you may look at the title of this chapter and argue the relevance is not apparent. Who, you may ask, decides what counts as knowledge and who chooses what knowledge is important?

Nursing, since the mid-twentieth century has been very concerned with its knowledge. Some of the debates have centred on the notion of professionalisation and the perceived need to identify nursing's unique knowledge base. Other aspects have been concerned with the focus of nursing's work: the person, and the need to identify what is important in terms of its impact on the person's health and illness experiences. In other words, what knowledge is important to enable nurses to make a difference?

This chapter offers a context in which to locate these debates. An outline of the history of philosophy and a consideration of the four main areas of philosophic inquiry provides such a context. It will allow the reader to identify significant influences on nursing and its development, and offer some insight into why we are where we are today. Because of the nature of this text, there is a heavier emphasis on the area of epistemology. This is not to undervalue the remaining areas of philosophical inquiry but indicates the emphasis in nursing to date.

INTENDED LEARNING OUTCOMES

By the end of this chapter you will:

1. be able to identify the main areas of philosophical inquiry
2. have an understanding of the history of knowledge
3. have explored your own conception of what it is to be a person and a nurse
4. begin to appreciate the significance of ethics and aesthetics for nursing
5. have some insight into the relevance of philosophic inquiry for nursing.

WHAT IS PHILOSOPHY?

Philosophy as it is referred to here relates to the academic discipline of philosophy as opposed to the philosophies commonly seen in clinical areas or nursing philosophies, such as those proposed by Nightingale or Henderson (Marriner-Tomey 1998). Philosophies seen in clinical areas are largely a statement of the values and beliefs of practitioners about care and the means in which care will be provided. They are linked to the academic discipline of philosophy in that statements such as 'we believe that all people are individual and entitled to be treated as such' are a verbal reflection of their underlying beliefs about the nature of people, which is one of the concerns of philosophy. What the practitioner may not have done is think about the origin and development of those beliefs. This is some of the business of philosophy.

Similarly, nurse theorists have proposed philosophies of nursing that are concerned with nursing and its purpose (Neuman 1995, Orem 1995, Roy 1984, Roy & Andrews 1999). Often these philosophies rest on the individual theorist's philosophical assumptions about people, knowledge or health. As Drevdahl (1999) claims, nursing ideas and theories have been developed, in the main, by women educated in Western institutions of higher learning and from diverse educational backgrounds who, therefore, bring their own perspectives to their writings. Thus they are said to be ideologically biased in that they are reflective of one person's view based on their own experiences. We need, then, to be able to analyse their ideologies against our own in order to identify if there is congruence.

Activity 1.1

Think of one value or belief that you hold.
Examine how you came to have this belief.
Justify your belief by offering reasons why you think this belief is right.

The immediate difficulty, of course, is that, if we have not explored our own beliefs about people, knowledge or health, we cannot hope to be able to analyse the conceptions of others. It is suggested here that this exploration can begin with philosophy.

In Greek, 'phila' means love and 'sophia' wisdom. Simply, therefore, philosophy can be said to be a 'love of wisdom'. The immediate difficulty with this definition is that there have been, according to Osborne (1992), sharp disagreements throughout history as to what constitutes wisdom. Similarly, there appears to have been much debate as to what constitutes philosophy, and the areas that have been addressed by philosophers since its inception in Greece in the sixth century BC have included, truth, reason, reality, knowledge, politics, language, ethics and logic, to name but a few. More recently, Karl Marx declared philosophy to be dead, and feminists have argued that philosophy is male dominated and a women's language must be invented to rethink it. Furthermore, Osborne (1992, 181) claims philosophy and science appear to have got us a 'huge environmental and political mess'.

Readers may ask what this has to do with the everyday world of nursing practice and how can philosophy help me when caring for people? In response, philosophy, it could be argued, reflects the socio-political concerns of the day. Philosophers' questions and answers, in any age, appear to have been governed by the world in which they lived. Therefore, it is suggested that, in order to understand the current world of nursing and where it may be going in the future, it is important to know from whence it came. Although it may appear to be stating the obvious, nursing is a product of the world in which it exists and it does not exist independently of that world. You may counter this argument by stating that sociological conditions can explain nursing's past, present and future, but in response it is worth asking what governs the sociological conditions, what drives political thinking, who makes the decisions and who has the authority to alter the course of a discipline such as nursing?

More importantly, who makes the decisions about what constitutes nursing and how it should be carried out? Rolfe (2000) argues that the question of power is central, where those who are *in* authority dictate, rather than those who are *an* authority, in determining what is considered important. A study of the history of philosophy highlights this point well if one considers what in philosophical terms is known as 'the Dark Ages'.

The rise of Christianity had a significant impact on philosophy in that it dominated it until the Renaissance. The power exerted by the Christian Church lay in its organisation and strength in an era where otherwise there was chaos. In establishing this power, the Church dictated the philosophical questions of the day. The previously liberal thinking was replaced by a more rigid system where freedom of thought was only tolerated if it was Christian freedom of thought (Osborne 1992). Philosophical concerns were largely replaced by religion, which had the answer for everything in the name of God. Philosophy thus became more metaphysical and concerned with the soul rather than with issues of ethics, politics or science. Likewise the dominance of the Christian Church in terms of philosophy waned, several centuries later, with a recognition of its corruptness, the horrors of the Inquisition and the rise of nationalism (Osborne 1992).

In order to illustrate these issues further in a nursing sense, a consideration of four customary areas of philosophical inquiry will be explored. Edwards (2001) identifies these as:

- epistemology
- ontology
- value-enquiry
- logic

EPISTEMOLOGY

According to Meleis (1991, 71), epistemology is 'the branch of philosophy that considers the history of knowledge. It raises and answers questions related to the origin, the nature, the methods, and the limitations in knowledge development and outlines the various criteria by which knowledge is accepted'.

The question of knowledge is as old as philosophy itself and the question 'what is knowledge' along with 'what is truth' was a major focus of early Greek philosophers, among them Aristotle and Plato. Osborne (1992) declares this early philosophical age was an extraordinary era of free thinking where the Greeks had started from the question of 'man's nature and his place in the universe' [sic] and constructed a whole method of reasoning out of it. Plato and Aristotle are credited with giving these modes of thinking a conceptual clarity and rigour that laid the foundations for future philosophical thinking. Aristotle was the first to attempt a classification of knowledge and these included:

- logic
- the categories
- metaphysics
- ethics
- politics
- biology
- poetics

The interesting fact about Aristotle was in the way history appeared to make him infallible, with his dogma remaining unchallenged in some areas for almost 2000 years. The Christian and Islamic faiths adopted many of his beliefs, and perhaps enabled those beliefs to be perpetuated and unchallenged.

At the end of the 'Dark Ages', referred to above, came the Renaissance, Reformation and Counter-reformation and began the phase of what is termed modern philosophy when the world was opened up to new thought. What is ultimately significant about this period is that it is largely associated with advances in science and the rise of the experimental philosophers. Although an oversimplification, this era was characterised by the development of the scientific method and the logic of induction (see 'Logic'). Furthermore, Descartes, known as the father of modern philosophy, proposed his 'Cartesian dualism' arguing essentially that the mind and the body are separate. The Enlightenment that followed was symbolised by continued advancement in science and the validation of knowledge through experience.

Enlightenment philosophers, usually referred to as empiricists, were epitomised by David Hume who claimed we should only trust those things that can be observed and measured and anything else is 'nothing but sophistry and illusion'. In the same way, John Locke saw the human mind as a blank piece of paper and believed knowledge of the world comes from experience alone.

The underlying belief throughout these periods of philosophical history was that there was an unalienable truth and that it was merely a matter of devising a method for accessing it. The trouble was that, with each development, flaws in the method for accessing this truth were subsequently highlighted. Flaws in the inductive method led David Hume to lose his faith in science. It also led another philosopher, Popper, to develop the hypothetico-deductive method, where the business of science was not to prove hypotheses but disprove them. Popper claimed that we could never know if we achieved the truth but theories that survived repeated testing could tell us if we had good grounds for believing we had discovered it.

However, in the twentieth century there was a subtle shift from the belief that there was an unalienable truth to what Thomas Kuhn (1970) referred to as truth dependent on rules and methods loosely denoted as 'paradigms'. Kuhn, a physicist, asserted that members of a scientific community subscribe to a paradigm, and accept its laws and rules about the focus of its work, the way problems are approached and resolved, and the manner in which its research is conducted. They tend to have collective beliefs and a common view of the world (world view). The important point here is that the paradigm itself is a 'given'. What the paradigm does is dictate methods and rules that serve to perpetuate it. A paradigmatic shift only occurs when the evidence is so strong that the community of scientists must change their conception of the truth. Paradigmatic shift occurs when the old methods no longer provide solutions to problems in the expected way. In the first instance, those who subscribe to the old paradigm initiate action to resist the new one. However, eventually the evidence is so strong that a shift occurs.

The implication of Kuhn's work was that there is no objective truth, but that truth changes according to paradigms employed for uncovering it. This has ultimately led to what Rolfe (2000) describes as a softening of the science of the enlightenment and the advent of what has been termed post-positivism, where subjectivity, even in physics, is being recognised. The history of the efforts to establish what it is to know has significance for nursing in the impact it had on what was and still is considered as important knowledge. Although some of the periods outlined above precede the formalisation of nursing, they had and continue to have an impact.

When Florence Nightingale declared her ideas on nursing, she attempted, according to Meleis (1991), to distinguish it from medicine by focusing on the environment and health as the concern of nursing. Subsequently, however, the goals of nursing became allied with those of medicine, in part because of medicine's more powerful and well-established position. Thus nursing programmes became focused on illness. Nurses adopted the language of medicine, and nursing complemented and perpetuated medicine's work. Moreover, medicine could be said to have been firmly entrenched in the scientific method, whereas aspects of environment and health as the concern of nursing did not 'fit' with what was considered to be knowledge or important knowledge. As these 'caring' aspects could not be articulated by employing induction, testing and generalising, they could not be verified as being valid.

A further facet relates to the earlier reference of the male-dominated philosophical and scientific world that is mirrored in the disciplines of medicine and nursing. The beginnings of modern nursing in the guise of Florence Nightingale and Mary Seacole in the Crimea, and Rofaida Al-Islamiah who accompanied the prophet Mohammed in his Islamic Wars are rooted in the identification by women of the need to care for the wounded. This firmly grounded nursing as the domain of women where care and comfort became the dominant ethic. Subsequent developments in the discipline have in some ways been hindered by these beginnings. Women are seen to be more affective, less scientific and altruistic, and the image of nursing is often one of mothering and nurturing. As Meleis (1991) states, Rofaida Al-Islamiah is regarded as the 'Mother' of eastern nursing, while Mary Seacole was referred to as 'Mother Seacole' by the troops in the Crimea.

Even in contemporary nursing, there is a belief that nursing knowledge is less defensible than medical knowledge. Nurses, at times, still appear to demonstrate an anti-intellectual bias. This is particularly reflected in the continuing discussions as to whether nursing should be an academic discipline. Nurses have argued that you do not need a degree to be a nurse, as it is essentially a practical discipline. Such a stance is significant in the support it has received from other women in media. For example, Nigella Lawson (*Observer*, 26th December 1996) stated that what is making students stay out of nursing colleges is Project 2000. This, she states, is 'the plan to make nursing more academic and theory based. And, frankly, can anything be more idiotic than that?' Pertinent to the chapter in this book, she expressed the wish that the nurse who looks after her in hospital has not majored in philosophy of nursing. Nevertheless, she does recognise that nursing can entail undertaking advanced medical techniques, but contends that intellectual ability is not a prerequisite for these and what nurses need is hands-on experience as shown in the accompanying picture to her article in which a nurse in traditional uniform is pouring a liquid into a funnel. What this article demonstrates is a lack of understanding both within and outside of nursing of what constitutes important knowledge for nursing. If we were to subscribe to the sentiments expressed in this article, nursing would forever be confined to the efficient performance of psychomotor skills.

The emergent question, then, is what is nursing knowledge? Much of the literature in the UK in the 1970s and 1980s was concerned with a consideration of whether nursing was a profession. Nursing began to consider itself as distinct from medicine and professionalisation was seen as one way of establishing that distinction. Although it is difficult to assess at what stage this became a goal of nursing, the twentieth century was seen as a time of great political and social change, and the emancipation of women, the Education Act of 1944, the establishment of the National Health Service and the World Wars were some of the more significant events. The process had begun much earlier in the USA, for example, Peplau wrote her Theory of Interpersonal Relationships in 1952.

The important requirement in terms of professionalisation was the development of a unique body of knowledge, in line with the traditional professions of the Christian Church, medicine and law. Although at this time there was a general dilution of what it was to be a professional, with the advent of professional footballers, builders, accountants and so on, nursing allied itself with the traditional professions and set about the task of identifying a body of knowledge, defining nursing, articulating what nurses do, why they were doing it and how to do it better (Drevdahl 1999). The argument was that, if nursing did not define its domain and the structure and content of that domain, then it would be difficult to articulate its knowledge base. As Clark and Lang (1992) point out, 'if we can't name it, then we can't control it, finance it, research it, teach it or put it into public policy'.

An important point worth mentioning here in relation to the focus of nursing's theoretical work was the decision to adhere to the rules and methods of the traditional sciences and medicine in terms of attempting to identify its unique body of knowledge. This could be said to be reflective of the power of the scientific method and what Rolfe (2000) refers to as the politics of desire. He goes on to state that

the modes of desire that nursing has submitted itself to for the last 150 years have been modes formed in our individual and collective unconscious needs to be like the 'other' to have what it is the 'other' has and which makes him legitimate and successful (Rolfe 2000, 96)

The 'other' in this case is medicine. Meleis (1997) has commented that when people look at a discipline through the lens of another discipline's domain, they tend to devalue and trivialise those phenomena and questions that may be central to it, but not to their own. This is what happens when nursing is seen, as it often is, through the lenses of medicine. Therefore, to adhere to the rules of medicine was somehow seen as a way in which to legitimise nursing and perhaps enhance its status.

Pierson (1999) argues the development of nursing science theory, nursing practice, education and research has been significantly influenced by Cartesian philosophy. In developing a distinct body of knowledge, nursing, using the conventions of Cartesian philosophy, would be able to describe, explain, predict and control the phenomena of concern in nursing practice.

Much of this work was undertaken in the USA where theorists such as Peplau, Orem, Roy and King began to articulate their conception of nursing. These early theorists drew on theories borrowed from other disciplines, for example, developmental theory (Orem), general systems theory (King) and adaptation theory (Roy), which Thorne et al (1998) state was consistent with the development of scientific knowledge at that time. The claim was that it is the way in which these theories are applied to nursing that identifies its uniqueness.

Fawcett (1984) in progressing this work proposed that the discipline of nursing should identify its parameters and areas of interest, and in doing so a general consensus within the discipline would be achieved. This is known as the metaparadigm of a discipline. She suggested that nursing had four metaparadigm concepts, and these are person, health, environment and nursing. Although these concepts are global it is proposed that 'scientists' (sic) within the discipline would have a general framework within which they could work. Conceptual frameworks subsequently developed by theorists within nursing using the metaparadigm concepts are seen by Fawcett (2000) as synonymous with paradigms. As is probably evident, this reflects Kuhn's discussion in respect of paradigms. By determining the parameters of the discipline, then the expectation is that its members will work within that paradigm adhering to its rules and its determination of what is acceptable and ultimately progressing the accepted view. Thus, in her subsequent publications, Fawcett has undertaken evaluation of conceptual models of nursing using these metaparadigm concepts as an indicator of the stage of development of the work. Those that are less developed in this area are seen to fall short of the expected standard. While this suggests a consensus, it is worth noting that several theorists have proposed alternative concepts of the metaparadigm (see Fawcett (2000) for further discussion). Nevertheless, such activity can be seen to be a way of legitimising and substantiating the discipline of nursing within the scientific community.

Likewise, the adoption of the nursing process and nursing diagnosis are seen by Pierson (1999) as a way of objectively and scientifically rationalising nursing actions (see Ch. 7). Nursing research was bound in measuring phenomena of interest and achieving generalisation about human conditions, all of which were consistent with working within the scientific method.

Until recently, then, the focus of nursing's epistemological work has been on knowledge acquisition and, while it would be easy to criticise the direction it has taken, it is suggested here that the reader must consider the contexts in which these developments happened. Moreover, as Whittemore (1999a) suggests, the scientific method, despite its limitations, has impacted and strengthened nursing.

Certainty and objectivity were challenged by Einstein's relativity, the principle of uncertainty as proposed by Heisenberg in 1924 and latterly quantum physics. Although it is outside the remit of this text to discuss these developments, the important issues are that they essentially questioned the belief that reality existed independently 'out there', that observation was the key to acquiring the truth and that objectivity in the observer was possible. However, these challenges to science came from within science itself. As Whittemore (1999a) states, they were not contradictory to classical laws but considered a different perspective, that is, probability rather than certainty.

Rolfe (2000) argues that a more fundamental criticism of science has come from outside science itself that not only questions the scientific method but the ends of science itself, and has been termed 'postmodernism'. Postmodernism in some sense could be said to represent the discontent with the perceived misuse of the power of science and evidence of the darker side of science. Whittemore (1999a) and Drevdahl (1999) argue these include global poverty, environmental degradation, worsening of health status for many, and continued atrocities in the name of ethnic and religious differences.

To simply define postmodernism is not possible and the reader is referred to Rolfe (2000) for a comprehensive discussion of its tenets or Klages (1997) (http:www.colorado.edu/English). However, a key feature of postmodernism is the tenet of an 'incredulity towards meta-narratives'. Lyotard (1979) (cited in Klages 1997) argues that society is governed by grand narratives or ideologies that are stories a culture tells itself about its practices and beliefs. In other words, a meta-narrative could be a story that is told to explain the belief systems that exist. An example would be the claim that democracy is the most enlightened form of government, and that it can and will lead to universal human happiness. In a culture that subscribes to the ideology of a democracy, rules and methods will be devised to protect that belief, activity will be directed at preserving the ideology and members of the culture in their living will emulate the belief.

Postmodernism, then, is a critique of these narratives. As Klages (1997, 4) claims, such narratives serve to 'mask the contradictions and instabilities that are inherent in any social organisation or practice'. Postmodernism favours 'mini-narratives' that are always contextual, temporary, and make no claim to generalisability, truth or reason.

Along with postmodernism has been the advent of feminist theory, which Sigsworth (1995) contends has relevance for nursing. Feminist theory advances the view that women's experience can be a legitimate source of knowledge and must be taken at its own merit rather than against the 'normed' male experience (Drevdahl 1999, 3).

In the nursing literature in the 1970s and 1980s, some opposition to the traditional scientific method in nursing began to emerge. Essentially, proponents of this view proposed that the scientific method could not explain the human experience (Leininger 1985) and that human science was more compatible with nursing and nursing values (Watson 1981). However, Gortner (1990), a proponent of the scientific tradition, cautioned against rejecting the scientific method out of hand and she suggested that it can be incorporated into a human science context. Such a stance could be supported, if nursing were to adopt a pluralistic approach whereby the scientific method could form one entity and other methods or approaches were equally valid in knowledge development. Some work like the seminal paper by Carper (1978) (see Ch. 2) began to lay claim to the other 'types' of knowledge as significant for nursing.

Since this initial work, there has been a gradual shift in the 1990s from knowledge acquisition as the focus of epistemology to one of understanding of the world in which nursing takes place. A significant contributor to this move has been Benner (1994) (see Ch. 2) and her commitment to an interpretive stance. Such a shift is concomitant with the branch of philosophical inquiry known as ontology.

Activity 1.2

Consider the word 'person' and reflect on what this conjures for you.
Having done this, write a description of a person. Do this as if you were trying to explain 'person' to an alien being who had never seen or would ever be likely to see a 'person'.
Now take time to consider the same question but substitute 'nurse' for 'person'.
When you have completed this, ask a member of your family or one of your friends to tell you what they think a nurse is. Give them time to consider their answer.

ONTOLOGY

Ontology, the theory of 'being', is part of the branch of philosophy known as metaphysics. Metaphysics deals with the nature of existence and, along with the theory of being, considers questions related to, for example, the origin and structure of the world. It is a characteristic of ontological questions to look at the defining features of an object. These questions have interested philosophers since its inception, but the depth and consideration of metaphysical issues has varied throughout history. Modern ontological debates stem, to a certain extent, from the work of Martin Heidegger, whose life work was the study of 'what is it to be a human being?' While Heidegger's philosophy is extremely complex and complicated, and his life history and work have been heavily criticised, Solomon (1985) claims his contribution to twentieth century philosophy has been significant.

Although it is not possible to even begin to outline Heidegger's work, what is significant for this text is his claim that the 'world' is constituted by and constitutive of the self. What he means is that the person is inseparable from the world in which they exist. Our world comprises a meaningful set of relationships, practices and language that we have by virtue of being born into a culture. He refers to our 'throwness' in the world, which means we are situated in a world that existed prior to our being in it (Heidegger 1982). The manner in which we compose our world is limited or constrained by language, culture, history, purposes and values (Leonard 1989). Persons are beings for whom things have significance and value, beings self-interpret and the person is embodied, that is, a 'being-in-time'. A significant notion is that the person can never be fully understood. There is no objective truth, and knowledge comes from persons who are seeking to understand others (Taylor 1994).

Heidegger has been attributed with initiating the existential movement in the twentieth century, although he denied the label. His work significantly influenced that of the French existential philosophers, Sartre and Merleau-Ponty, and tenets of his philosophical claims can be said to be present in contemporary postmodernism and feminism. Postmodernists reflect the view that the self can never be universal, neutral or static, and feminists speak of the need for multiple voices and multiple truths (Drevdahl 1999). Drevdahl (1999) also claims the current debates about the concerns of nursing in terms of person reflect the philosophical concerns of postmodernism and feminism.

As discussed in the previous section, person is conceived as one of the meta-paradigm concepts of nursing. Theorists put forward their conception of the concept person and in doing so lay claim to a particular philosophical view. For example, Edwards (2001) highlights four conceptions of person, namely:

- persons are biological organisms
- persons are composed of mental and physical properties, but the former cannot be reduced to the latter—a dependence view
- persons are essentially mind or souls
- persons are 'body subjects' in which mind and body are inseparably 'intertwined'.

Each of the above views can be found in the work of various nursing theorists. The first view that persons are biological organisms can be found, according to McKenna (1997), in the work of Henderson (1966). This view reflects the biomedical view of the person where all states are attributable to physical phenomena. The second view is evident in the work of Roy (1980) and is sometimes known as token identity theory (Edwards 2001, 75). In this view the mental properties are dependent upon physical ones but cannot be reduced to them. The third view can be found in the work of Watson (1988), who considers that mind and body are essentially independent and reflects the Cartesian dualism referred to earlier. Lastly, Benner and Wrubel (1989) and Parse (1998) reflecting the work of Merleau-Ponty (1962) propose that the body is an instrument of the soul where the soul or brain is the person. In this view, 'the whole of the body and the person comprise the same entity' (Edwards 2001, 79).

It is not the intention here to explore the merits and weaknesses of each view [for this, the reader is referred to Edward's (2001) text] but to highlight the complexity of the question of 'what is a person?'

It is unquestionable that the nature of persons is central to the practice of nursing, since persons are the focus of its work. It is also proposed that one's view of 'person' will influence how nursing is practised and will dictate, to a certain extent, what is considered to be health and, by association, what is illness. Similarly, the therapeutic strategies adopted will arise from these original conceptions.

For example, if we subscribe to the view that a person is a biological organism, then it implies that all health problems are physical and illnesses of the mind are attributed to the physical. Thus, illness is identified by physical examination and treatment regimes are essentially physical. Conversely, if we believe that persons are essentially mind or souls, then we consider that these are separate entities (Cartesian dualism) and health problems can arise either in the body or the mind. Therefore, treatment regimes are directed towards either the body or the mind. Adherence to the Merleau-Pontian view that the mind or body are inseparable means that all health needs have physical and mental components, and all treatments thus focus on both. Edwards (2001) contends this view would argue against the divisions between, say, adult and mental health nursing. Finally, the dependence view argues that health needs can arise in either the physical or the psychological, and so treatments could be directed at either. The important distinction between this view and that of the biological organism stance is that the mental cannot be reduced to the physical.

Activity 1.3

Consider the four views of person outlined above.
Try and outline what you think might be the weaknesses of each view.
Take each view and attempt to apply it to a patient who has been diagnosed as being in a persistent vegetative state.
What do you think would be the implications for the treatment of this patient?

Having previously considered your own view of person and those outlined by Edwards (2001), you may have identified that it is derived, in part, from your experiences and beliefs. These may have been located in your personal experiences and beliefs bound in the family, society and culture in which you live, or may have arisen from your nursing experiences. It is proposed here that, whatever your views, they will have a moral dimension. For instance, your view of person will have been influenced by the morals of your family, your culture and society, and nursing. In turn, your view of person will impact on your moral decision-making in practice. This is significant as Edwards (2001, 112) claims nursing can be understood as a moral response to human vulnerability and is thus an 'essentially moral enterprise'.

VALUE-ENQUIRY

The main components of value-enquiry are ethics and aesthetics. Ethics, according to Beauchamp and Childress (1994, 4) 'is a generic term for various ways of understanding and examining the moral life'. Ethics can be classified as normative ethics, descriptive ethics, metaethics and philosophical theory.

Carper (1978, 20) in her paper argues that ethical knowledge is a pattern of knowing in nursing. An appeal to ethics is necessary in a discipline where fundamental questions arise about morally right or wrong action in connection with the care and treatment of illness and promotion of health. She goes on to claim that nurses require an understanding of different philosophical positions regarding what is good, what ought to be desired and what is right as well as having knowledge of ethical frameworks to deal with complex moral judgements and what obligations a nurse has by virtue of possessing that title. Schröck (1990) refers to this as 'knowledge why' and will be explored in greater detail in Chapter 2.

Most nurses are familiar with normative ethics, which Beauchamp and Childress (1994) claim is a twentieth-century notion. Normative ethics attempts to provide norms for the guidance and evaluation of conduct. In nursing this is evident in the production of a particular Code of Professional Conduct that appeals to general norms, such as not harming others, respecting autonomy, maintaining confidentiality and so on. However, it is suggested here that an appeal to a code of conduct may not always help a practitioner in a situation that requires a moral judgement about practice. Pattison (2001, 8) goes so far as to suggest that codes of conduct do not necessarily 'develop or support the active independent critical judgement and discernment that is associated with good moral judgement and, indeed, good professionalism'. Therefore, Carper's position that an understanding of philosophical theories and ethical frameworks is necessary is supported in that the skills associated with being an autonomous 'ethical practitioner' requires more than knowledge of codes.

Contemporary philosophical theories can be located in the study of ethics by philosophers since the Greeks. For example, ethics was a major concern of Socrates who stated 'the unexamined life is not worth living' and he was deeply concerned with morality and with discovering the just, the true and the good (Osborne 1992). Over the succeeding centuries, various philosophers have proposed theories that are largely concerned with how people should behave. Virtue-based or character ethics is based on the writings of Plato and Aristotle while natural law derives from the writings of the Stoics. Utilitarianism was proposed by Jeremy Bentham in the eighteenth century and developed by John Stuart Mill in the nineteenth century. Deontology is based upon the ethical thought of Immanuel Kant and is now more commonly known as Kantian theory.

Aesthetics, the study of art and beauty, has significance for nursing and is located in the claim by some that it can be described as art. Carper (1978) and Peplau (1988) both support the contention that nursing is an art and a science. To a large extent, nurses unquestionably accepted this claim as it provided an explanatory and justifying framework for those activities or attributes considered 'good nursing', but that could not be described as science in the traditional sense. However, Carper's claims are being questioned specifically in reference to the claim of aesthetics in nursing (Edwards 2001, Wainwright 2000). Edwards (2001) argues that Carper appears to conflate the ideas of art and skilled performance of a craft.

A study of aesthetics as a branch of value-enquiry, while not resolving the issue of nursing's art, does offer some insight into the debate. For example, what do nurses mean when they use the term 'art'? Are they referring to the traditional Greek and Latin terms of 'ars' and 'techne', which refer to skilled activity, or are they laying claim to nursing as 'fine art' as in painting and poetry?

Edwards (1998) believes nursing is not a 'fine art', while Carper (1978) presents a case for expanding the definition of fine art to include nursing. Wainwright (2000) believes this was erroneous and argues for a broader understanding of aesthetics after Dewey (1934). Dewey believed that it was not necessary to expand the definition of fine art but rather extend the notion of aesthetics into non-artistic activities. Therefore, according to Wainwright (2000), his notion supports the contention that there can be an aesthetic appreciation of nursing but not that nursing is a fine art.

The need for clarification is bound in the potential confusion this could create amongst nurses. As with all aspects of nursing, its writers have a particular stance or view. If such views are inarticulate, then it poses difficulties for judging what constitutes nursing's art (see Ch. 2 for a more detailed discussion).

LOGIC

The final branch of philosophy to be discussed in this chapter is that of logic. Logic according to Edwards (2001) is not concerned with details of specific arguments, but rather the process or form of such arguments.

As with much of philosophy, logic has its beginnings in the work of Socrates, Plato and Aristotle. According to Johnson and Webber (2001), Socrates initiated his followers into a method of cognitive reasoning known as the Socratic Method. This method was largely concerned with question and answer, and involved questions such as 'why', 'what', 'what if', 'explain', 'justify' 'what do you mean' and 'how do you know'. Socrates' task was to persuade his followers to rationalise their vague, unsupported thoughts.

To some extent, reasoning through inquiry has changed little and nursing uses this method to explore nursing phenomena. Reasoning in nursing asks for justification of one's thoughts and opinions and, in doing so, the nurses access a variety of sources to substantiate their claims (see Ch. 7).

Knowledge developed through reasoning must conform to the rules of logic, which Chinn and Kramer (1999) state is either deductive or inductive. Deductive reasoning was originally founded in the work of Aristotle, who perfected the system and termed it 'syllogism'. It works thus:

Premise: All men are mortal
Premise: Socrates is a man
Conclusion: Socrates is mortal
(Osborne 1992)

As is demonstrated in deductive reasoning, a conclusion follows from one or more statements that are taken as true. Changing either of the premises or changing the conclusion without changing one or more of the premises is known as faulty reasoning. Deductive reasoning is commonly taken to be specifying from the 'general' to the 'specific'. It is a process of knowledge development where the theory comes first and is, therefore, also known as 'a priori' reasoning. Following the development of the theory, research is undertaken and the end result is a theory that is either accepted, rejected, modified or needs further testing. McKenna (1997) states Einstein's theory of relativity is a particularly good example as the theory was developed many years before the methods were available that could test it.

In contrast, inductive reasoning specifies from the 'specific' to the 'general' and is known as 'a posteriori' reasoning. To demonstrate this, McKenna (1997) offers the above example but applied inductively:

Premise: Confucius is a man and is mortal
Premise: Socrates is a man and is mortal
Premise: Hannibal is a man and is mortal
Conclusion: All men are mortal.

The idea is that enough observations are made of phenomena that share a common characteristic until a confident generalisation can be made. Induction has been the method favoured by the empiricists as it relies on observation or experience of empiric reality and traditionally is located in scientific thought. However, contemporary nursing integrates non-traditional or phenomenological thought, and qualitative research methods can use induction to generate knowledge from practice (see Ch. 4).

Both inductive and deductive reasoning are features of clinical reasoning, evidence-based practice and models of decision-making. Reasoning according to Johnson and Webber (2001) is more than just critical thinking. It involves an integration of traditional scientific thought and non-traditional or phenomenological thought (see Ch. 7 for further discussion of critical thinking and decision making).

Johnson and Webber (2001) also introduce the notion of abductive reasoning. This type of reasoning or logic involves using propositions that have no proof. It is about making a conceptual leap based on experiences, observations and beliefs to form an 'educated guess' about the phenomena in question. Although the proposition will have to be tested subsequently, the basic premise is that this form of reasoning in nursing allows for the inclusion of the influence of experiential learning on nurses' judgements. Writers who support such a view of nursing include Belenky et al (1986), Benner (1984), Benner and Wrubel (1989) and Carper (1978), and are explored in more detail in Chapter 2. The immediate difficulty, however, is in articulating those judgements in a health-care arena where accountability for one's actions demands explication, as, for example, in evidence-based practice.

Therefore, logic offers processes by which theories can be generated and tested through research. Logic also offers structures for examination of clinical reasoning and allows for the development of other processes, such as that of abductive reasoning.

SUMMARY

In summary, this chapter has offered a brief insight into the development of philosophical thinking, and its direct and indirect influences on nursing. The discussion of the four main areas of philosophic inquiry demonstrates how nursing has been concerned with its epistemology and the development of a unique body of knowledge. The exploration highlights that these issues are not resolved nor is there any real consensus about how they should be progressed.

There is, however, evidence of a philosophical shift towards a consideration of ontological questions related to what it means to be a person. These are attributable to the influence of postmodernism and feminist thinking on nursing, where it is contended that there is no objective truth, but multiple truths and multiple means for accessing them.

The discussion on value-enquiry incorporating ethics and aesthetics highlighted their significance for the practice of nursing. The conception that nursing is essentially a moral enterprise located in the vulnerability of human beings emphasises the centrality of ethics. Aesthetics is an area of exploration that is significant in considering nurses' art.

Finally, a study of logic underlines the significance of understanding reasoning in nursing as it forms the basis of justification for action.

Many of the issues raised in this chapter will be discussed in greater detail in the succeeding chapters, beginning in Chapter 2 with an exploration of the concept of knowledge and knowledge in nursing.

2

How do we know?

INTRODUCTION

This chapter attempts to articulate some of the debates regarding knowledge in nursing. Much of the contemporary discussion in the nursing literature centres on what is considered important knowledge for the discipline. This has been led, to a certain extent, by the view that the western traditional view of knowledge, 'knowledge that' or propositional knowledge, does not account for all the knowledge needed by the nurse in clinical practice. Although a consensus has not been achieved as to what counts as important knowledge for nursing or even the types of knowledge used, key texts by Carper (1978), Benner (1984) and Belenky et al (1986) are presented in this chapter in order to locate the debate for the reader.

Prior to exploring their work, a necessary overview of 'what is knowledge' or 'what counts as knowledge' is presented. While the discussion is by no means exhaustive, it highlights the complexity of the concept and the inherent difficulties with articulating 'what is knowledge'.

INTENDED LEARNING OUTCOMES

By the end of this chapter you will:

1. have explored your own conception of what it is to know
2. be able to offer an example of a model of knowledge
3. be able to distinguish between propositional and practical knowledge
4. have an understanding of Carper's (1978) fundamental patterns of knowing

5. be able to relate Benner's (1984) six areas of practical knowledge to your own area of practice
6. be able to identify with types of 'knowers' in nursing in respect of the work of Benner (1984) and Belenky et al (1986)

Activity 2.1

Consider something you know (it does not have to be nursing related) and write it down.
Now think about *how* you know it and write down your rationale.

KNOWLEDGE

Nursing literature over the last 20-30 years is full of papers related to nursing knowledge and its development (Fawcett 1995, 2000, Gortner 1990, Meleis 1985, 1991, 1997), its uniqueness (Benner 1984, Carper 1978), its structure (Fawcett 1989, 1995, Fawcett et al 2001), its relationship with research and theory (Meleis 1985, 1991, 1997, Silva 1977), and its constituents in terms of types (Benner 1984, Carper 1978, Chinn & Kramer 1991, 1995, 1999), to mention but a small sample.

Of particular significance to this chapter is the work of Carper and Benner. Carper in 1978 proposed that the body of 'knowledge that' serves as the rationale for nursing practice and has 'patterns' named as 'empirics', 'esthetics' (sic), 'personal' and 'ethics', while Benner and Wrubel (1982) and Benner (1984) began the process of differentiating 'theoretical' (knowledge that) from 'practical' (knowledge how) knowledge. While these aspects have been explored in considerable depth, few nurse writers, including Carper and Benner, have articulated what they mean by 'knowledge' and 'what it is to know'.

Chinn and Kramer (1999, 1), have defined knowledge in that they propose 'knowing' to refer to 'ways of perceiving and understanding the self and the world'. They see knowing as a dynamic and changing process. 'Knowledge', they claim refers to 'knowing that is in a form that can be shared or communicated with others'. Although this definition has changed slightly in its wording from previous editions of their work (1991, 1995) it is easy to see why Edwards (2001) has argued it is vulnerable. If interpreted, as he does, that perception equals knowing, his claim is justified from the point of view that perceptions can be erroneous and such perceptions communicated and shared with others cannot be classed as knowledge (see discussion below for knowledge criteria). To illustrate his point, Edwards (2001) offers an example of the perception that when viewing rail tracks in the distance they appear to converge. That they do not converge justifies his view that perception cannot be classed as knowledge.

However, if the view is taken that 'perceiving and understanding' cannot be separated in Chinn and Kramer's (1999) definition, then the interpretation that perceiving equals knowing alters. According to the *Chambers English Dictionary* (1995), to understand is to 'grasp with the mind the meaning, nature, explanation or implication of'. Therefore, knowing does not simply occur as a result of perception but through the process of understanding. Whittemore (1999b, 365) appears to agree when he refers to knowledge as 'a highly sophisticated integration of the experience of the moment with the processes of the mind'. If we then return to Edwards' example of the erroneous perception of rail tracks converging in the distance and apply understanding, we would be aware of the misperception through our ability to grasp the meaning of the occurrence and we would 'know' that rail tracks do not converge.

Despite the addition of understanding, the continuing vulnerability in Chinn and Kramer's (1999) definition is that there is potential for what is communicated to others (knowledge in their view) to be erroneous. However, they go on in the text to qualify their claims by stating that 'knowledge represents what is collectively taken to be a reasonably accurate account of the world as it is known by the members of the discipline' and knowledge 'is a representation of knowing that is collectively judged by standards and criteria within, in this instance, the nursing community' (Chinn & Kramer 1999, 2). Therefore, the accuracy of the account of the world must be judged by a set of criteria. What Chinn and Kramer do not do is offer criteria or conditions for judging whether something can be regarded as knowledge.

Johnson and Webber (2001) also consider the concept of knowledge but in contrast to Chinn and Kramer they distinguish knowing from understanding. They take the view that 'knowing' is merely 'being aware of' and you can know or have knowledge without understanding. For example, a person can know that the normal range of body temperature is between 36°C and 37°C, but may not understand its significance or why it is so. However, they do argue that there is a relationship between knowing or knowledge and understanding in that you cannot have the latter without the former. For instance, you cannot understand the normal range of body temperature unless you know or have knowledge of it.

Ultimately, their definition is vulnerable since the distinction between knowing or knowledge and understanding appears to centre on what could be classed as levels of knowledge. To take the example above, surely not understanding the significance of the normal range of body temperature is related to a level of knowledge rather than the difference between knowledge and understanding.

What this brief discussion highlights is the complexity and difficulty with articulation of the concept of knowledge. If you return to the activity above and consider your rationale for knowing something, you may have listed some criteria for justifying your claim. Within the sociology of knowledge, several models have been proposed in order to identify criteria for judging whether something can be regarded as knowledge.

KNOWLEDGE CRITERIA

Scheffler (1965, 21) proposed a tripartite model of knowledge containing the conditions of 'truth', 'secure belief' and 'evidence'. In this model, knowledge is defined as a justified true belief (Edwards 2001, 26). The 'truth' condition claims that, if a person 'knows' something, they must not be found to be in error. The 'belief' condition insists that, if a person 'knows' something to be true, they must also believe it to be so and, lastly, the evidence condition states that there must be some evidence to support the claim of what is known. In this model all three conditions must be met. Edwards (2001) claims that what this model clearly identifies is that, for a belief to count as knowledge, there must be some evidence. To some extent this counters claims to intuition as a source of knowledge where a person may say 'I know something is wrong' but may not be able to offer any evidence of why they believe this, and so their belief does not meet the criterion for knowledge.

According to Edwards (2001), it is preferable to base our actions on what is known rather than what is believed, as it provides firmer ground. Usually when we claim to know something we begin by believing it to be so. However, the degree of certainty with which we hold the belief can vary. For example, have you ever attended a quiz where you are a member of a team and, despite your belief that you know the answer, you have allowed your team to convince you otherwise? If you recall why you allowed this to happen, you may conclude that it was to do with your level of certainty about your belief. You may say, 'I think I am right but I am not very sure'. If it subsequently transpires that your answer was correct, your degree of certainty is enhanced or, conversely, if you are shown to be incorrect, you revise your belief.

If we propose then that certainty is a prerequisite for knowledge, we could arrive at a position where it could be claimed that we cannot possess any knowledge at all since absolute certainty is not possible. As Descartes claimed, our senses sometimes deceive us and, therefore, nothing is as it appears, and we can never be sure we are not dreaming (Osborne 1992). Quine and Ullian (1978) support the tenet that absolute certainty is not possible when they suggest that any statement or theory can be subject to revision. However, they propose that beliefs can be counted as knowledge by adopting criteria (virtues) for judging their plausibility. These virtues are:

- conservatism
- modesty

- simplicity
- generality
- refutability

(Quine & Ullian 1978)

In order to demonstrate how these virtues can be applied in determining how plausible a belief is, we will use the following example. In respect of wound cleansing, there was considerable debate in the late 1980s–early 1990s about the benefits of using antiseptics. Antiseptics were determined to have toxic effects following experimental research on animals and their use had to be weighed against any possible advantages. While all antiseptics were included, most discussion was centred on the use of Eusol (Dealey 1999).

The first virtue of conservatism requires that we do not readily accept new beliefs that would mean surrendering previously held beliefs that were seen as successful. The use of antiseptics, including Eusol, could be said to have been a plausible belief given their ability to destroy vegetative compounds, including bacteria, by preventing their growth. Furthermore, the use of antiseptics contributed to the widely held belief that the wound must be kept clean and dry. Thus, the new belief that antiseptics were potentially harmful was met with disbelief. The strength of the desire, particularly by doctors, to hold on to the previous belief is evidenced by published papers calling for clinical trials (Leaper 1992) and accusations of naivety against nurses who were being 'manipulated', it was claimed, by manufacturers of dressings.

The second virtue concerns the modesty of the new belief. We are less likely to accept a new belief if it requires an alteration to our whole set of previous beliefs. However, if it were likely only to require a modification or adjustment, then we are more likely to accept it. To a certain extent advocating the cessation of the use of Eusol in wounds does not meet the requirement of modesty. The new belief required considerable alteration to a belief that had been in effect since World War I, where Eusol was used on heavily infected wounds. Thus, the challenge could not have been said to be a modest one.

Simplicity is the third virtue and states that the simpler the belief, the more likely it is to be plausible. In our example the previously held belief has the appearance of being simpler given the associated widely held belief about the purpose of antiseptics. The challenge demanded that we accept that antiseptics are potentially harmful and, therefore, does not meet the simplicity virtue.

The fourth virtue is one of generality and is concerned with how widely the belief can be applied. Therefore, a piece of research that produces results that can be applied to the whole population rather than a particular group within the population is seen to be more desirable. This virtue is often used as a key indicator in determining the value of a piece of research. The evidence for cessation of the use of Eusol was primarily undertaken on animal studies and could be said to have been a general theory in that it applies to all mammals. Thus the virtue of generality could be said to have been met.

Nevertheless, the resistance to the new belief about Eusol was bound in the final virtue of refutability that concerns attempts to test the new claim. However, some claims cannot be tested. In our example, there were calls in the medical press for clinical trials concerned with refuting the claim about Eusol. If this meant using Eusol on some patients, then it is questionable whether such a practice would have been warranted from an ethical perspective.

As can be seen from our example, the challenge to the use of Eusol meets the virtues of generality and refutability, but it does not meet those of conservatism, modesty or simplicity. Taken thus, it would seem that the claim is less plausible than a claim, say, that meets all the virtues. This could be said to be the weakness of such a model given that, in our example, the new belief was ultimately accepted and Eusol is no longer used in the cleansing of wounds. The evidence to support the new claim was such that adherence to the previously held belief was no longer viable. Furthermore, a claim could be made that not all virtues can be considered 'equal', and maybe those of generality and refutability are more significant in determining what counts as knowledge.

The final point is that this model clearly demonstrates that all beliefs cannot be on an equal footing. Some beliefs are more easily changed or challenged than others. Quine (1980) proposes a framework for this conception of knowledge, which he refers to as a 'web of belief'. At the centre of the 'web' are those beliefs that are not easily challenged while those at the periphery are more likely to change.

This discussion has centred on what Kuhn (1970) and Polanyi (1958) consider to be 'knowledge that' or propositional knowledge, which is bound in a traditional western view and where the emphasis is on abstract reasoning. The central tenets are that theory comes before practice and, in the performance of an activity, the person simply applies the knowledge they have to the skill in hand.

PRACTICAL KNOWLEDGE

The challenge to the claim that all knowledge is propositional arises from both tenets. In nursing this can be located mainly in the work of Benner (1984) who considered the distinction between propositional knowledge (know that) and practical knowledge (know how). Benner's conception of know how is bound in the clinical experience of the nurse or, as she claims, 'the knowledge embedded in clinical practice' (Benner & Wrubel 1982, 11). The basic argument is that propositional knowledge does not account for the knowledge required to, say, give an injection or record a blood pressure. While a person can learn the theory of giving an injection or recording a blood pressure, that does not mean that they will be able to do so. Recording a blood pressure involves feeling for a pulse, listening for the Korotkoff (thudding) sounds that cannot be known by simply knowing the steps in the performance of the procedure. Think when you first had to record a blood pressure. Most nurses will note the difficulty they had locating the radial and/or brachial pulse and thereafter 'hearing' the Korotkoff sounds. It was only with experience that the performance of the skill became more fluid. Merleau-Ponty, a French philosopher (cited in Reynolds 2001) refers to this as 'bodily knowledge', where it is not only the mind that possesses knowledge, but knowledge can be located and possessed by the body.

Benner and Wrubel (1989) argue that practical knowledge is not just confined to the performance of motor skills, but includes nonverbal, interpersonal communication such as looks, posture, gestures and actions like touching. This is discussed further in the section on Benner.

Secondly, the nature of nursing dictates that practice comes before theory. As Peplau (1952) argued, knowledge development in nursing begins with observations made in the context of practice. Therefore, the theory before practice aspect of propositional knowledge does not account for this. Edwards (2001) inserts a note of caution into the casual acceptance of the notion of practical knowledge. He claims a nurse cannot just possess practical knowledge—it must be in relation to a particular skill or area of practice. Secondly, the person must be able to perform the skill successfully in order to be said to have practical knowledge. Therefore, the poor performance of a skill cannot be classed as practical knowledge.

This section has given a necessarily brief insight into the concept of knowledge. The next section will explore some of the key areas of knowledge development in nursing focussing particularly on Carper's patterns of knowing, Benner's conception of practical knowledge and a brief consideration of the significance of Belenky et al's (1986) women's ways of knowing for nursing.

CARPER'S FUNDAMENTAL PATTERNS OF KNOWING

Carper's (1978) paper on nursing's patterns of knowing has had a significant impact on the discussions about nursing knowledge. Although Carper specified these patterns should be seen as the whole of knowing, they are, for the purposes of description, reduced to: 'empirics', the science of nursing; 'esthetics' [sic], the art of nursing; the component of personal knowledge in nursing, and ethics, the component of moral knowledge in nursing (Carper 1978, 14).

Empirics—the science of nursing

Empiric knowing according to Chinn and Kramer (1999, 4) and after Carper (1978) is expressed in practice through the nurse's scientific competence. The knowledge itself comprises theories, facts and laws that have been developed through traditional scientific methods (Carper 1978). These methods involve hypothesis testing in a context-free and objective manner for the purpose of explaining, prescribing and predicting phenomena of special interest to nursing. For example, germ theory, which began with the work of Louis Pasteur and was progressed by Robert Koch and Joseph Lister, still directs the use of aseptic techniques in all aspects of surgery and wound healing.

According to White (1995), Carper's conception of the science of nursing is limited. This is because it is located in the time when she undertook her work and when the scientific approach referred to in Chapter 1 was dominant. As a result, there is little consideration of knowledge developed in ways other than the traditional scientific approach. White (1995) argues the definition of empirics should be expanded to accommodate contemporary nursing science where knowledge developed using other methods such as phenomenology, ethnography and grounded theory (see Ch. 4) is valued. These methods are not concerned with creating general laws, but about enriching understanding of the human experience and are a valid focus for nursing science. Thus, the merit of a theory is found in its practical implications and usefulness in solving problems in the discipline. Therefore, as Reed (1995) claims, the empirical includes the practical.

According to Chinn and Kramer (1999), empiric knowledge is created through processes of explaining and structuring, and replication and validation. Explaining and structuring involve the two processes of creating conceptual meaning, and structuring and contextualising theory.

Creating conceptual meaning 'produces a tentative definition of a concept and set of tentative criteria for determining if the concept exists in a particular situation' (Chinn & Kramer 1999, 57). For example, if you wanted to study the concept of reassurance in your area of practice, you would first have to define what you meant by reassurance. In the process of doing so, you would develop some criteria or indicators in order that you can ultimately judge whether the concept existed in the area of study. This activity is not arbitrary but systematic, and commonly used methods for creating conceptual meaning include concept clarification, concept analysis and concept development (see Ch. 5 for a discussion of these).

Structuring and contextualising theory is concerned with forming systematic links between and among concepts, resulting in a formal theoretical structure (Chinn & Kramer 1999) or, put more simply, it is about constructing a theory. All theories comprise concepts, and theory construction is concerned with establishing the relationships between these concepts. Theory construction is a highly complex activity and approaches will vary depending on whether you are constructing a new theory or whether you are developing somebody else's previously constructed ideas (see Chs 3 and 4 for further discussion).

The replication and validation of empiric phenomena are achieved through the relationship between theory and research. Research provides the vehicle for validating or testing theory. What is important in terms of nursing is that a variety of research methods other than the traditional scientific method can be employed, depending on the nature of the question and the stage of conceptual and theoretical development (see Ch. 4 for a more detailed discussion).

Aesthetics—the art of nursing

Both Carper (1978) and Peplau (1988) claim nursing lost sight of its art in the pursuit of its science. The value of Carper's work, according to Fawcett et al (2001) is that she expanded the historical view of nursing as an art and a science. In the past, nursing's artistic element has been associated with both domestic (mothering and homemaking) and nursing (procedures including comforting) arts, and latterly as an art form similar, but not identical, to the performing arts (Peplau 1988).

Carper (1978) sees aesthetic knowing as expressive and is not amenable to description in language. Its expression is in the art act itself. It is made visible, according to Chinn and Kramer (1999, 6), through 'the actions, bearing, conduct, attitudes, narrative and interactions of the nurse in relation to others'. The action of the nurse involves a perception of the patient's behaviour so that the need being expressed by the patient can be determined. Aesthetic knowing is about moving beyond the surface, to sense meaning and connect with the unique human experience of the other (Chinn & Kramer 1999).

Carper sees empathy as being an important mode in the aesthetic pattern of knowing. The more experience the nurse gains in empathising with the lives of others, the greater her repertoire of choices in designing and providing nursing care that is effective and satisfying.

As mentioned in Chapter 1, both Edwards (2001) and Wainwright (2000) perceive difficulties with Carper's apparently interchangeable use of 'art' and 'aesthetics'. Wainwright (2000, 754) claims that 'most accounts of fine art and aesthetics differentiate between the art object produced by the artistic process and the subsequent aesthetic appreciation of it'. Put more simply, fine art concerns production and aesthetics involves appreciation. Carper appears to include both of these in her discussion on aesthetics. In her view, the performance of the nursing act equates with the artistic process, thus forming the basis for her claim of fine art. The subsequent action of the nurse in meeting the patient's need appears to be the basis for claiming an aesthetic quality where there are possible criteria for evaluating the performance of the nurse, for example, the repertoire of skills used.

The question to be posed here is: does it matter whether nursing is considered a fine art or possesses aesthetic qualities? The tentative answer is that there seems to be a general agreement in the literature as to the existence of nursing art (Johnson 1994) but little consensus as to what that means. Whether you believe the interchangeable use of 'art' and 'aesthetics' by Carper is merely semantics (Tschudin & Hunt 1998, van Hooft 1998) or not (Edwards 2001, Wainwright 2000), the issue is in the various interpretations and the potential for confusion for learner and practising nurses. For example, Chinn and Kramer (1999) and Silva et al (1995) argue for nursing as a fine art, while others primarily focus on the notion of practical know-how that includes any skill or technique that a person has in a particular situation (Hampton 1994, Johnson 1994). Until some clarification is reached, then criteria for judging 'nursing's art' remain elusive. Benner's (1984) work in this area is significant and will be discussed in the next section.

Personal knowing

Personal knowledge according to Carper (1978, 18) is concerned with 'the knowing, encountering and actualising of the concrete, individual self'. She goes on to state that 'one does not know about the self; one strives simply to know the self'. Personal knowing, she proposes, is the most difficult pattern to master and teach. It cannot be expressed in language and can only be described as the self that *was* through reflection, stories and autobiographies. Even in this form, the self can never be truly known to others.

Carper claims that, without personal knowledge, therapeutic use of self is not possible in the interpersonal encounter. Personal knowing is about the self and self-awareness, and the processes of coming to know the self. Personal knowing involves creating congruence between the authentic self and the self as disclosed to others. It is only through knowing the self that we can hope to know others and, through that, knowing can accept ambiguity, difference and vagueness (Chinn & Kramer 1999, White 1995).

The importance of personal knowing is about the development of an authentic personal relationship between two people. Fundamental to this relationship is reciprocity.

Ethical knowing

In this pattern of knowing referred to as ethical knowing, Carper (1978, 21) stated 'the examination of the standards, codes and values by which we decide what is morally right should result in a greater awareness of what is involved in making moral choices and being responsible for the choices made'. Ethical knowing then is concerned with 'matters of obligation or what ought to be done' (Carper 1978, 20). As stated in Chapter 1, Carper asserts that it is more than just knowing the ethical codes of a discipline and includes all actions that are subject to a judgement about whether they are right or wrong.

Schröck (1990) refers to this as 'knowledge why'. She states it is not enough to possess 'knowledge that' and 'knowledge how', but each act should be undertaken on the basis of whether it ought to be done. A practitioner may know how to undertake a skill and may possess the attendant knowledge, for example, of anatomy and physiology, but the decision about whether it ought to be done with the ultimate aim of benefiting the patient is a moral question.

She continues that moral reasoning must be based on a rational foundation, and an ability to articulate one's moral position in a coherent and logical way. This she states is achieved through enquiry into moral perceptions, moral reasoning and moral argument, and essentially constitutes an examination of self, thus supporting White's (1995) view that moral knowing and personal knowing are closely linked. Such exploration safeguards against the moral desensitisation that Schröck proposes is a feature of the novice's socialisation into a profession. Benner (1984) and Benner and Wrubel (1989) propose that such learning can take place effectively through an exploration of practice using reflection, critical analysis, storytelling and discussion.

The rationale for utilising practice as the arena for moral enquiry is based on Carper's contention that the complexity of ethical issues in the health-care field means that an appeal to ethical theory and codes may not provide universal answers. An appeal to theory or the 'rulebook' may provide some basis for rationalising decisions in moral dilemmas but, as Carper highlighted, the nature of practice means that moral choices must be made in relation to the specific situation and in the context in which they happen.

Furthermore, Benner (1984) and Benner and Wrubel (1989) contend the practice arena provides a milieu for discerning the moral ideal of what is good, rather than what is just. The notion of doing what is good can be said to be located in the belief that traditional models of moral reasoning reflect a predominantly male orientation. Gilligan (1982) claims that men see morality in terms of rights and justice, whereas women view it in terms of care arising from attachments to others and a very strong sense of being responsible.

Before moving on to discuss the influence of Benner's work on conceptions of nursing knowledge, some final points regarding Carper's work are presented. Carper clearly outlines that 'each pattern may be conceived as necessary for achieving mastery in the discipline but none of them is sufficient' (Carper 1978, 22). Chinn and Kramer (1999) believe that knowledge within any one pattern must be critically examined and integrated into the whole of knowing. Failure to do so, they claim, leads to distortion, narrow interpretation and partial use of knowledge instead of understanding. For example, Schröck's (1990) claim that 'knowledge that' (empirics) and 'knowledge how' (aesthetics) have brought the world to the brink of nuclear destruction, and where medical expertise has and is still being used to torture and kill people efficiently, demonstrates the potential for abuse of knowledge when it lacks consideration of 'knowledge why' (ethics).

Finally, some thought must be given to the view that Carper's work is not fixed or cannot be challenged. Silva et al (1995) claim Carper's work is located in an epistemological era and does not incorporate the philosophical shift to ontological concerns (see Ch. 1).

White (1995) believes there is potential to add another pattern of knowing to Carper's original work that should be entitled 'socio-political knowing'. She claims the other patterns of knowing address the 'who', 'what' and 'how' of nursing practice, while socio-political knowing identifies the 'wherein'. It concerns the socio-political context of the nurse and the patient, and the socio-political context of nursing, including the society's understanding of nursing and vice versa.

Munhall (1993) also proposed a fifth pattern of knowing referred to as 'unknowing'. Munhall sees 'unknowing' as an art, although Heath (1998) contends that the focus of the exploration appears to be on personal knowing. Unknowing seems to be related to an awareness of the possible negative impacts of not remaining open to other possibilities. Heath (1998) proposes, therefore, that unknowing is related to all four patterns of knowing. Unknowing is about recognising the gaps in one's empirical knowledge, being aware that there are ethical dilemmas that cannot be solved, and recognising the possibility that being an expert can foster rigidity and an assumption that there is no more to be learned. Without unknowing, negative habitual practice, where the practitioner is confident in his or her knowing and is closed to new learning opportunities, is a potential danger.

Finally, it is suggested that, although Carper's work had enormous significance for nursing knowledge development, nurses are cautioned against an uncritical acceptance of her views.

BENNER—NOVICE TO EXPERT

The main focus of this section primarily concerns Benner's (1984) *From Novice to Expert* text, although references to subsequent publications are included.

While Benner does not use the term 'art' in her writing, her conception of practical knowledge or know how contains elements associated with the art of nursing. She contends that 'experience' is a prerequisite for the development of expertise, but that it is not merely the passage of time or longevity. Experience as she uses the term 'results when preconceived notions and expectations are challenged, refined or disconfirmed by the actual situation' (Benner 1984, 3). She claims that expertise in human decision-making makes the interpretation of clinical situations possible, and it is the knowledge embedded in this clinical expertise that is central to advancing nursing practice and science. She claims the problem-solving skills of the expert nurse differ from those of the novice and such a difference can be attributed to experience.

Benner (1982, 4) identified six areas of practical knowledge, and claimed these must be articulated in order to identify and extend clinical practice. She identifies these as graded qualitative distinctions, common meanings, assumptions, expectations and sets, paradigm cases and personal knowledge, maxims and unplanned practices.

Graded qualitative distinctions are concerned with comparing judgements in nursing situations as examples present themselves. It is about defining and refining descriptive language in order to communicate with each other and achieve consistency. For example, when recording a patient's pulse, descriptive language can be employed to grade or qualitatively distinguish the 'feel' of the pulse, through employing terms such as 'pounding', 'thready', 'strong', 'weak' and 'erratic'. Only through articulating and communicating these judgements can consistency be achieved.

Activity 2.2

Think of other examples from your area of practice where you might use descriptive language similar to the example above.

Common meanings according to Benner (1984) form a tradition. Nurses, over time, develop these common meanings about their practice and the people who are the focus of their practice. Common meanings can become apparent through narrative accounts of diverse clinical situations. An example of how articulation of patient experiences can lead to common meaning is Herth's (1990) study that explored the concept of hope in terminally ill patients (see Ch. 5 for activity related to hope).

Activity 2.3

Consider some common meaning you and your colleagues have in your area of practice that has an impact on your subsequent practice.

Practice and practice situations are laden with assumptions and expectations derived from observation and experience of working with similar and dissimilar patients. Sets are concerned with a predisposition to act in a particular way in a given situation. We would argue here that practising nursing with certain assumptions, expectations and sets could impact negatively on practice. For example, if a nurse is working from a particular 'set' related to assumptions and expectations of a particular patient group, that will determine how she behaves in that situation. A pertinent example is a patient who consistently requests his analgesia at the exact time it is due. One nurse could be bound in the assumption that the patient is 'becoming addicted'; another might believe that such behaviour is an indication of the inadequacy of the analgesia. Benner (1984) believes critical incident analysis is a useful strategy for identifying divergent practices.

Activity 2.4

Identify an example from your area of practice where a set can:
• negatively impact on patient care
• positively impact on patient care.

A paradigm case is one in which the clinical lesson stands out in bold relief (Benner & Wrubel 1982, 15), and can alter the practitioner's subsequent understanding and perception of future clinical situations. Articulation of paradigm cases are useful tools for teaching students of nursing because they convey more than principles and guidelines. They communicate the whole situation. However, Benner (1984) suggests some paradigm cases cannot be clearly articulated as their significance is in the interaction between the given situation and the practitioner's previous knowledge that creates 'the experience'. This personal knowledge is defined by Benner (1984, 9) as 'the personal history, the intellectual commitment and the readiness to learn that the practitioner brings to the clinical situation. It is the interplay between this personal knowledge and the situation that determines the subsequent actions and decisions'.

Activity 2.5

Reflect on your practice and try to identify one experience that impacted significantly on your subsequent practice.
Attempt to articulate its significance.

Maxims are simply 'cryptic' instructions that only make sense if a deep understanding of the situation already exists. For example, a coronary care nurse may indicate subtle rhythmical changes in a patient's cardiac status that will only make sense to another who has experience of observing cardiac patients. To the novice, maxims can appear unintelligible. Benner (1984) argues that expert nurses can learn from sharing maxims with each other, but that they are also a useful learning tool for the less expert nurse as it can help them gain clues about clinical knowledge.

Activity 2.6

Try to think of an example of a maxim from your clinical practice that you now understand but previously did not.
Outline how you came to understand it.

Finally, Benner (1984) refers to unplanned practices as those that have, through changes in health-care systems and delivery of health care, become the domain of nurses. Examples would include taking on activities previously in the domain of the doctor. She argues that taking on such roles alters the nurse's clinical judgement and perceptions, and should, therefore, be studied to identify the 'know how' that develops in their practice.

Activity 2.7

If you undertake a role that was previously the domain of the doctor, consider how it might have altered your perceptions of practice or influenced your clinical judgement.

Benner argues that these six areas of practical knowledge can be observed in the expert nurse. In order to articulate the notion of an expert nurse, Benner (1984) applied Dreyfus and Dreyfus' (1980, 1981) (cited in Benner, 1984) model of skills acquisition to nursing. Dreyfus and Dreyfus propose that there are five levels of proficiency in the acquisition and development of a skill, namely novice, advanced beginner, competent, proficient and expert. Benner, in applying the model, used the terms skill and skilled practices synonymously, and did not limit it to particular psychomotor skills, but included skilled nursing interventions and clinical judgements.

The novice has no experience of the situation in which they are expected to perform. Because of their lack of experience, they are given rules to guide their performance. Novices are limited in their ability to read 'whole situations' and tend to focus on tasks that do not require experience of the situation. Novices are learner nurses entering a new clinical area but can also be nurses who transfer from their previous area of expertise. Therefore, the model of skills acquisition is a situational model. For example, learner nurses, who may have learned how to record a patient's blood pressure but have not carried out the skill in a clinical setting, will focus intensely on the performance of the activity. It is likely that they will not attend to other aspects of the patient's situation.

Advanced beginners are those who have experienced enough real situations to be able to recognise aspects of the situation. Prior experience is necessary for aspect recognition, which encompasses an appreciation of the global characteristics of a situation. For example, the advanced beginner may begin to recognise features of, for instance, pain behaviour in a patient. However, this would be dependent on having previous experience of observing a patient in pain. The advanced beginner still depends on rules and needs support in the clinical setting to help with aspect recognition.

The competent practitioner is one who has been in practice for two or three years in similar situations. Competency implies an ability to discriminate between what is most important in a given situation. Competent practitioners use analysis and conscious deliberate planning that helps achieve efficiency and organisation. They demonstrate some elements of mastery, but do not function with the speed and flexibility of proficient practitioners.

The proficient practitioner is one who sees situations as wholes rather than a series of discrete aspects. In a positive sense, the proficient practitioner with the attendant experience comes to know what to expect in given situations and by association is able to distinguish when it does not occur. The proficient practitioner has well-developed decision-making skills and is able to discriminate quickly where the problem exists. According to Benner (1984), proficient practitioners use maxims that reflect the nuances of the situation.

Expert practitioners no longer rely on rules, guidelines or maxims to link their understanding of the situation with the correct action. Here, Benner refers to the notion of 'intuitive grasp' when delineating the practice of the expert nurse. Expert nurses focus on the accurate area of the problem without wasteful consideration of alternative diagnoses and/or solutions. That is not to say experts never use analytical tools, as in some situations they may not have had previous experience or may simply have grasped the situation incorrectly. Experts' performance is fluid and flexible, and to some extent the practice becomes part of the practitioner in that they are not consciously practising.

Having delineated Benner's views, it is considered important to note that they are not without their problems. Primarily, there appears to be a lack of clarity as to how she considers propositional knowledge in relation to practical knowledge. According to Johnson (1996, 173), Benner, along with others, considers that the use of 'scientific knowledge to determine an appropriate course of action inhibits the perfection of nursing practice', as it precludes a holistic grasp of a given situation. If taken literally, this claim could imply that perfect nursing practice places little emphasis on propositional knowledge.

This implication arises from the sometimes expressed view that 'intuition', a term that has been attributed to Benner, is itself a basis for action. It is worth noting that Benner uses the term 'intuitive grasp' rather than 'intuition'. The difficulty with such an interpretation is that actions based on intuition alone are not rationally defensible, particularly in a discipline such as nursing that is accountable for its actions. The alternative interpretation is that the expert nurse sees whole situations, where subtle cues based on empirically available data prompt intuitive judgement. At the time of action, they may not have been able to articulate the process, hence the phrases 'it was a gut feeling' or 'a feeling', but on reflection were able to identify cues that prompted the subsequent action. This interpretation is supported in Benner's (1984) exemplars of expert nurses recounting significant events or experiences.

Furthermore, if we adopt the view that expertise is based on experience alone, then there is the potential for practice to become entrenched in the view of the expert. How then will revisions to propositional knowledge be incorporated into the expert's practice? By adopting the term 'expert' there is an implicit assumption that their actions constitute 'good' practice. What constitutes good practice changes as revisions to knowledge occur (see the Eusol example in the earlier section 'Knowledge criteria'). Therefore, expert nurses, in order to remain 'expert' must achieve a fusion of 'knowledge that' and 'knowledge how' and, as referred to in the previous section, remain open to the possibilities of new learning.

Rolfe (1997) proposes there is a level beyond expertise or expert, as described by Benner. It is characterised by mindful practice and informal theory building, uses reflection-in-action after Schön (1983) (see Ch. 9) and is referred to as reflexive practice. The reflexive practitioner applies 'mindfulness' to every individual aspect of their work by formulating and testing hypotheses, and informally building theories about the individual situation as it manifests. Thus, the potential negative aspects of practising habitually or routinely inherent in Benner's notion of expert are negated.

Activity 2.8

Consider the discussion on Benner's model and attempt to place yourself on the continuum from novice to expert in terms of your current area of practice. Offer some rationale for your decision.

WOMEN'S WAYS OF KNOWING

The inclusion of women's ways of knowing, after Belenky et al (1986), is based on the notion that there are some parallels between women's ways of knowing and nursing (Kidd & Morrison 1988, Meleis 1991, Nelms & Lane 1999, Schultz & Meleis 1988). Women's ways of knowing, according to Nelms and Lane (1999), is a feminist epistemology that rejects traditional notions of knowledge and knowledge accumulations. They also believe women's ways of knowing offers a model for understanding the more discursive kinds of critical thinking reflective of the moral integrity essential to nursing. Belenky et al (1986) classified women along a continuum from silent to constructed knowing that reflect women's views of knowledge, truth and authority. Meleis (1991) and Schultz and Meleis (1988) proposed that these types could be found in nursing. Below is an outline of the five types with some tentative suggestions for possible connections to nursing using Meleis.

Silent knowers are those who are unable to trust their own experience as knowledge (Belenky et al 1986). Those in authority are all knowing. Silent knowers have no voice. According to Meleis, these knowers in nursing know their practice but are unable to theorise or articulate their knowing. Consequently they are invisible.

Received knowers interpret information literally. Learning is receiving and retaining, and occurs by listening and being told. Received knowers depend on and value the expertise of others. These knowers do not believe that the work they produce is as valuable as that produced by others. They tend to quiet their own voice in order to listen to others. This, Meleis (1991) claims, is reflected in the way nursing has bought into and accepted without question theories and paradigms, or is evidenced by nursing's unthinking acceptance of the dominance of medicine.

Subjective knowers according to Belenky et al (1986) are those who believe there are still 'right answers', but value their own voice and experience as sources of knowledge. Truth is an intuitive reaction—'something experienced rather than actively pursued or constructed' (Belenky et al 1986, 69). These knowers believe in multiple personal truths but fear offering opinions that may conflict with others. Authority is associated with power and is to be mistrusted. Meleis (1991) believes these knowers in nursing can produce 'knowledge that', which informs nursing in ways that no other knowledge can. She likens the knowledge these knowers produce to personal knowledge after Carper (1978) and expert knowledge after Benner (1984). However, given the discussion above about Benner's expert nurse and the susceptibility of these knowers to a fear of offering opinions that may conflict with others, caution must be exercised in accepting Meleis' interpretation.

The procedural knowing category has two positions of separate and connected knowing. Procedural knowers see the process of making decisions as more important than the decision itself. These knowers speak with the voice of reason. Some truths are truer than others. In this category, separate knowing comprises a detached adversarial stance. There are clear procedures for establishing truth. This knower is autonomous, but suspicious that anyone and everyone may be wrong.

Connected knowers use reciprocity and remain connected to others even when there is disagreement. These knowers enjoy collaborative working. Nelms and Lane (1999), in their study, claim there is a maturation process where nurses can move from the position of separate knower to the perceived more mature position of connected knower. Belenky et al (1986, 121) claim connected knowing is just as procedural as separate knowing, except the procedures are not so clearly coded and defined. Meleis (1991) believes these knowers are the rationalists in nursing and are those who communicate rules, procedures and regulations. Thus, she believes these knowers are best suited to developing empirical theories. This may be the case for separate knowers but it is questionable whether it applies to connected knowers.

Finally, constructed knowers are those who listen to their own voices as well as others. These knowers are able to integrate separate and connected knowing as the interaction demands. Knowledge is tentative and under-standing occurs from considering knowledge in context. They see them-selves as creators of knowledge and value various strategies for knowledge development. According to these knowers, all knowledge is constructed and the knower is an intimate part of the known (Belenky et al 1986). Meleis (1991) claims these knowers believe that knowledge development is constant and always in process. They accept that situation and knowledge are contextual and subject to differing interpretations.

As with Benner's novice to expert, women's ways of knowing can be seen as a useful development tool for individual practitioners. For example, Nelms and Lane (1999) used Belenky et al's (1986) schema to determine student nurses ways of knowing and found that over time they matured along the continuum towards connected knowing. Kidd and Morrison (1988) also used Belenky et al's work to explore the similarities between the growth processes of women and theory development in nurs-ing. However, further work is needed on the usefulness of women's ways of knowing for contemporary nursing. For example, do the parallels between women's ways of knowing and nursing encompass men in nurs-ing? Do men in nursing adopt women's views of knowledge, truth and authority? As stated earlier, Gilligan (1982) argues that women's moral development is distinct from that of men's. Women, she claims, tend to an ethic of care and responsibility, while men tend to an ethic of rights and jus-tice. She acknowledges that these types of development are not gender exclusive and reflect a tendency. Nonetheless, there are several interesting questions that may be worthy of investigation. For example, do men enter nursing because they reflect a care ethic traditionally associated with women and nursing? Do they reflect a rights and justice ethic that may reflect a differing perspective to what might be the dominant view? Does any difference in ethic cause a dissonance for male and female nurses working together? Although these questions are speculative, they highlight the care needed in subscribing to an epistemology that could potentially ignore a significant percentage of nurses.

Activity 2.9

Using Belenky et al's continuum, consider what type of knower you are in relation to your clinical practice.
What are the reasons for your decision?

SUMMARY

This chapter has considered the concept of knowledge in relation to nurs-ing. The complexity of the concept was highlighted particularly in terms of determining what is considered knowledge and what it is to know. Criteria for judging whether something can be regarded as knowledge were presented using the tripartite model of knowledge, and Quine and Ullian's 'virtues'. It was noted that there is no absolute certainty in respect of what is considered knowledge, and no statement or theory cannot be subject to revision.

This discussion focused on the traditional western view of knowledge, namely propositional knowledge. A challenge to propositional knowledge was presented concentrating mainly on Benner's claim that it does not account for the knowledge embedded in clinical practice, that is, practical knowledge.

The work of Carper and Benner comprised a major focus in the chapter in view of the significant influence of their work. Carper's (1978) seminal paper on fundamental patterns of knowing in nursing was presented with a brief critique in light of developments in contemporary nursing. Benner's six areas of practical knowledge were explored and her contention that these can be seen in the 'expert' nurse examined. Her model for skills acquisition, novice to expert, was discussed and a brief overview of possible problems with the model was offered.

Finally, Belenky et al's (1986) women's ways of knowing was included in light of the proposition that, as a feminist epistemology, they have significance for nursing. Using Meleis, some tentative suggestions of the existence of these 'knowers' in nursing are offered, although it is acknowledged that the interpretation is subject to challenge.

Overall, the important issues in this chapter are concerned with a challenge to the view that propositional knowledge accounts for all knowledge. In contemporary nursing, there is a ready acceptance that nursing incorporates other types of knowledge, and non-traditional methods for accessing or constructing knowledge of importance are being accepted. Furthermore, there is a belief that nursing has an artistic element, although the debate continues as to its nature. These points encapsulate the significance of the work of nurse writers such as Carper and Benner. However, the final point cautions the reader against an uncritical acceptance of their views given the earlier point that there is no certainty and no knowledge is absolute.

3

What is nursing theory?

INTRODUCTION

The previous chapter was largely concerned with knowledge and types of knowledge used in nursing. Although knowledge and theory are not synonymous, they are related in that theory provides knowledge about the world. Theory structures the generation of knowledge deemed to be important to a discipline as well as providing direction and organisation. It is this relationship with knowledge that gives it its inherent value.

According to Timpson (1996, 1030), 'nursing theory has a reputation for abstraction, even irrelevance in the minds of many practitioners'. To some extent this is not surprising given the numerous meanings assigned to the term 'theory'. Some, for example Landers (2000), refer to it to mean the subject matter taught in the classroom, while nurse theorists themselves do not agree as to what is or what is not theory, with a resultant confusion for any practitioner being introduced to its world. Furthermore, the abstract and complex terminology fuels the conception that theory is far removed from the reality of practice, thus resulting in practitioners disregarding it as irrelevant.

The purpose of this chapter, therefore, is to attempt to unravel the world of theory. The chapter is necessarily limited and selective given the plethora of literature and books on theory and nursing. It is important to acknowledge at this point that there exist numerous definitions of theory, and what is presented here is interpreted from the available literature. That is not to say it is definitive, and reading other texts may highlight different interpretations. Ambiguity does exist and, for those studying nursing theory, tolerating such ambiguity is part of the process of coming to an understanding of its world. However, while not disagreeing that theory can be and is taught in the classroom, the manner in which the term is employed in this chapter does not refer to the subject matter of the curriculum. The discussion will begin by an exploration of 'what is theory?' before going on to examine 'what is nursing theory?'.

INTENDED LEARNING OUTCOMES

By the end of this chapter you will:

1. be able to offer a definition of theory in your own words
2. understand that what is considered theory varies according to the definition
3. understand terms such as 'phenomena', 'idea', 'concept', 'proposition' and 'hypothesis'
4. be able to identify and explain one framework associated with 'levels of theory'
5. have examined the attributes of each level of theory
6. be able to offer examples of each level of theory.

THE WORLD OF THEORY

Activity 3.1

Think back to conversations or dialogues you have had and consider whether you have ever said, 'I have a theory'.
Think of the situation in which you said it and write down your 'theory'.
Make some notes about the features of your theory.
(Note: it is not important at this point whether your 'theory' can actually be defined as such, as this exercise is about defining characteristics of theories).

We will begin this section by highlighting that there are multiple definitions of theory. Despite the differences, all appear to have some common characteristics, the first of which is that theory is concerned with some aspect of the world. Theory does not, however, necessarily describe reality, but speculates on how it might be or how it ought to be. Thus, theories are always subject to change, they are not absolute and always exist in uncertainty (see Quine & Ullian in Ch. 2 regarding certainty in knowledge).

To illustrate this point in the sixteenth century, Copernicus challenged the static medieval view that the earth was the centre of the universe and proposed that the earth orbited the sun. While this is now a generally held conception and has been verified to the extent that it is the currently accepted knowledge or truth, at the time, this proposal was met with derision and generally rejected. The power over acceptance or rejection of theory at the time rested firmly with the Church in Rome, and what was seen to be acceptable theory or truth was determined by it. Therefore, the world view or paradigm (see Ch. 1) was one that subscribed to Aristotelian principles. The most notable follower of Copernicus between 1543 and 1600 was Galileo, and such was the power of Rome that he was summoned by the Inquisition to stand trial for 'grave suspicion of heresy' for supporting Copernicus' theory. As a consequence, until the late seventeenth century, those who supported Copernican theory did so in secret (Westman 2002).

While some theories may eventually have a universal impact, generally they tend to be grouped together and focused on aspects of the world that are of interest to a particular discipline. For instance, most people will have heard of Einstein's theory of relativity and we may even know a little of what it is about. Yet it is unlikely that most of us will understand or even see the relevance of the theory. It almost certainly would not appear to have any impact on our daily lives. However, for mathematicians, physicists and scientists, Einstein's theory has had an enormous impact in terms of attempting to explain aspects of the world (its structure) in which they are particularly interested.

Conversely, if we examine developmental theories like those proposed by Piaget and Erickson, we would be more likely to grasp the relevance. We know, for example, that children's development is judged against the milestones in developmental theory, and thus they have wide and universal application.

Another common characteristic of theories are phenomena. Phenomena according to Johnson and Webber (2001, 14) are the basic building blocks of theory and are 'observable and researchable connections between objects, events or ideas'. Meleis (1991, 12) states phenomena are 'all aspects of reality that can be consciously sensed or experienced'. Phenomena are so called because they comprise two or more objects, events or ideas that are in relationship with each other. For example, you may observe that a patient who has had surgery may be moaning and/or crying and sighing, grimacing, guarding and/or lying perfectly still. Prior to giving a name to this occurrence, you are noting a phenomenon, which remains just that prior to any cognitive interpretation (McKenna 1997).

Johnson and Webber (2001) also refer to 'noumena', which are similar to phenomena but are perceived rather than directly observable. Examples include the relationship between culture and pain behaviour, spirituality and health, and intuition and decision making. Most writers appear to group phenomena and noumena together, and refer to a continuum of phenomena from concrete and observable to abstract and intangible.

Phenomena, when labelled, are referred to as concepts (Johnson & Webber 2001, McKenna 1997, Meleis 1997). Labelling phenomena offers some classification or categorisation, and attempts to convey their meaning or their properties. Therefore, concepts are not in themselves a real entity but are a tool. In our example of the post-operative patient, the verbal and non-verbal behaviour of the patient could be labelled as a response to post-operative pain or pain behaviour. Concepts offer a more efficient and concise way of communicating.

With a slightly different emphasis, Chinn and Kramer (1999, 54) define concepts as 'complex mental formulations of experience'. By experience they mean perceptions of the world such as objects, people, sound, colour, inter-actions and so on. What is important here is the notion of perception. Because of perception, which is in turn influenced by a person's beliefs, values, background and culture, two people may give differing conceptual labels to the same phenomena. Moreover, the same word may be used to convey several different meanings and can be on a continuum from concrete to abstract.

Activity 3.2

Consider the word 'key'. Write down the various ways in which the word is used to represent different kinds of objects or ideas.
Now indicate which ones may be regarded as concrete and those that are abstract.

You may have written 'key' to represent:

- an instrument used to turn a lock, wind a clock, grip and turn a nut
- a series of buttons or levers on an instrument to sound musical notes
- a button to display a character on a computer, typewriter or calculator
- a pitch or tone of a voice, for example, 'low key'
- a system of musical notes related to each other in a scale
- a central idea in presenting an argument or discussion
- a means of achievement

(*Chambers English Dictionary* 1995)

You may have noted that some usages of the word 'key' convey the image of an object (an instrument used to turn a lock), while others (a means of achievement) are symbolic and, in turn, are either concrete or abstract in terms of whether they can be directly observed or only be experienced indirectly. Therefore, the use of a concept is context bound (see Ch. 5).

We can see, then, that an individual concept can vary from the concrete to the abstract, but there is also a continuum of concrete to abstract for all concepts. While concepts such as cup, key, chair, and table may appear at the more concrete end, there are those that are more abstract. Some of these are used in nursing, such as trust, hope, reassurance, anxiety and empathy, to name but a few. Concepts that are highly abstract have a less concrete reality base and are sometimes referred to as 'constructs' (Chinn & Kramer

1999, McKenna 1997). However, constructs are often made up of less abstract or more observable concepts. An example of a construct could be 'self-esteem' (McKenna 1997).

While Johnson and Webber (2001) regard phenomena as the building blocks of theory, most writers refer to concepts in this way (Becker 1983, Chinn & Kramer 1999, Fawcett & Downs 1992, King 1988, McKenna 1997).

Regardless of whether phenomena or concepts are seen as *the* building blocks of theory, the important point at this juncture is that theories comprise statements about relationships between concepts and these are written in the form of propositions. Johnson and Webber (2001) also refer to propositions as relational statements, while Fawcett and Downs (1992) distinguish between propositional statements that are either nonrelational or relational (see Ch. 4 for further discussion). Propositions, then, are another feature of theories. A proposition identifies the nature of the relationship between the concepts. According to Chinn and Kramer (1999), a proposition is a general term that includes a number of different types such as postulates, premises, suppositions or assumptions, axioms, theorems and hypotheses.

Assumptions and suppositions are taken to mean the same and concern aspects within a theory that are taken for granted or thought to be true without empirical evidence or testing, usually because they are reasonable (Chinn & Kramer 1999, McKenna 1997). According to Meleis (1997), they often reflect values, beliefs or goals. If we take our post-operative patient who is demonstrating pain behaviour as an example, we might take it for granted that it is surgery rather than a particular type of surgery that results in pain behaviour, or assume that pain is harmful for a patient.

Postulates and premises are similar and are used in deductive logic as the basis for forming a conclusion (see Ch. 1 on deductive logic). Examples of premises are hypotheses and axioms. Axioms are used for deducing theorems, especially in mathematics. Hypotheses are statements that tentatively suggest a relationship between two or more variables that can be tested. Conclusions and theorems are products of deductive logic with the latter being confined largely to mathematics and physics.

At this point, let us illustrate the exploration thus far by using the example of the post-operative patient. In your clinical practice you observe that patients who have had surgery demonstrate behaviour that may include moaning and/or crying and sighing, grimacing, guarding and/or lying perfectly still (phenomena). You may label this phenomenon pain behaviour (concept). In this instance, you develop the proposition that surgery causes pain behaviour.

The question that arises at this point is whether you now have a theory. The answer is that it depends on how theory is defined. As mentioned in Chapter 1, the members of a scientific community subscribe to a paradigm or world view, and accept its laws and rules about the focus of its work, the way problems are approached and resolved, and the manner in which its research is conducted. Thus, they also adopt the definition of theory that fits with that paradigm. For example, the scientific method values measurement, objectivity, refutability and generalisation. Therefore, theories developed and ultimately accepted as valid within this paradigm must meet these criteria. An example of a theory definition that equates with the criteria is that of McKay (1969, 394) who sees theory as 'logically interrelated sets of confirmed hypotheses'.

Essentially, what this definition implies is, if a theory is not testable, then it cannot be given the label 'theory'. Furthermore, as prediction and control are inherent in this view, theory testing usually involves quantifiable empirical research studies. Through testing and retesting, theory develops knowledge and ultimately becomes 'established theory' in the form of facts, principles and laws (Johnson & Webber 2001).

Chinn and Jacobs (1987) suggest that much of what is described as nursing theory does not meet these criteria, and Maquis Bishop (1989) questioned whether nursing theory even exists, that is, whether there is theory that exists that is unique to nursing, not whether nursing uses theory.

Johnson and Webber (2001) refer to theories that are not established theory as 'speculative theory'. Much of nursing theory could be said to fall within this bracket, if we consider the dearth of evaluation and testing. Alternatively, and as proposed by Dickoff and James (1968, 198), the definition of theory could be expanded to incorporate that which is established theory as well as speculative or theory in development. To this end, they proposed a definition of theory that stated 'a theory is a conceptual system or framework invented to some purpose'.

Chinn and Kramer (1999, 51) have also developed a more encompassing definition of theory that they identified as 'a creative and rigorous structuring of ideas that projects a tentative, purposeful and systematic view of phenomena'.

These definitions do not state that theory is an 'anything goes' process, but is purposeful and invented for some purpose. The important distinction from McKay's definition is that they do not require a hypothesis to be tested before a statement can be regarded as a theory. Thus, in respect of these definitions, nursing theory exists but does so at different levels.

Activity 3.3

Think about your practice and try to identify theories you use in your speciality.
Now try and fit these theories with one of the above definitions.
Could the theories you have identified be tested by research?
How do you think they could be tested?

Prior to discussing levels of nursing theory, a final point regarding theory is worth mentioning. Regardless of the definition of theory, in order to determine if it fits reality (say the reality of clinical practice) and is, therefore, useful, ultimately reality must be consulted (Dickoff et al 1968). Reality is consulted through the vehicle of research. Theory provides knowledge about the world in which we live through research.

NURSING THEORY

For the purposes of this section, Walker and Avant's (1995) framework for levels of theory is used to structure the discussion. That is not to say others do not exist but Walker and Avant's is widely used and accepted as a logical structure. The levels of theory as identified by Walker and Avant (1995, 5) are:

- metatheory
- grand theory
- middle range theory
- practice theory.

Each of these will be defined and explored and their place in nursing's theoretical development established.

METATHEORY

According to Walker and Avant (1995), metatheory is concerned with the broad issues related to theory in nursing. Metatheory considers philosophical and methodological questions related to the development of nursing's theory base. McKenna (1997) refers to metatheorists as 'theory watchers'. Some of those who have been classified as metatheorists include Dickoff and James (1968), Fawcett (1984, 1989, 1995, 2000), Meleis (1991, 1997) and Walker and Avant (1983, 1995) to name but a few. Over the last 30–40 years the metatheoretical debates have focused on:

- What is nursing and what is not nursing, what are the concerns of nursing?
- What has philosophy got to do with nursing?
- What has nursing theory got to do with basic science theory?
- Is there one universal theory or framework that answers all of nursing's questions?
- How do we do our research in nursing? What are the best methods to be employed that reflect our concerns about the practice of nursing?

Many of these issues were referred to in Chapters 1 and 2, and they constitute the business of metatheorists. The significance of their work may not be immediately apparent in everyday practice but their indirect influence is in how they highlight contemporary issues of importance for debate within the discipline. In highlighting the issues, they encourage us to consider how we want nursing to be now and in the future. Walker and Avant (1995) claim there is a reciprocal relationship between metatheory and other levels of theory. Metatheory, through analysis of broad nursing-theory issues, clarifies the role and choice of method for the other levels of theory development. In turn, the other levels of theory provide material for further analysis and clarification at the level of metatheory.

An example of the impact of the work of metatheorists is evidenced by the work of Dickoff and James (1968), who, with colleagues, proposed a more encompassing view of theory (see p. 46) than that of the dominant scientific paradigm. They also proposed a description of the nature of theory in a practice discipline such as nursing as well as how it could be developed. This will be discussed in more detail under 'Practice theory', but the point here is that their proposal stimulated intense discussion and, to a certain extent, gave nurses permission to shift away from traditional science when considering their theoretical development.

A further important point for readers is that metatheorists do not necessarily agree among themselves on the broad issues of concern in nursing. Meleis (1991) and Timpson (1996) argue that this lack of agreement is acceptable in an emerging discipline such as nursing where, as part of the process of evolution, competing views, acceptance and rejection, and reconsideration should be tolerated. It is merely an indication, they claim, of nursing's status as a 'would be' discipline.

However, Engstrom (1984) has argued this lack of consensus has to some extent created confusion among nurses. If learner or novice theorists cannot make sense of the debates, it only serves to put them off pursuing further understanding.

At a very fundamental level, metatheorists do not agree on what can be defined as theory. Some subscribe to a traditional view of theory and argue that, unless a theory can be tested, it cannot be regarded as such (Fawcett 2000, Uys 1987). In this view, then, what are commonly described as nursing models are seen to be concerned with broad issues in nursing and, as the concepts within them are at too high a level of abstraction for testing, they are not theories. Others, like Meleis (1991), subscribe to a broader definition of theory, and believe that theory can exist at a number of levels and that testing is not a prerequisite. In this view, nursing models are classed as grand theories.

This point is made because students, on reading various theory texts, will encounter both views and will ask 'which one is right?' The answer is that some understanding of the rationale for both positions should be achieved and, thereafter, the choice is personal. There are persuasive arguments in both positions but, as Meleis (1991) and Stevens-Barnum (1994) claim, it is the content that matters, not what we call things.

GRAND THEORY

For the purposes of this chapter, what are termed nursing models or conceptual frameworks are incorporated under the heading of grand theory. After the sociologist Merton (1968), grand theory is defined as highly abstract and broad in scope. When referring to scope, it means the breadth of possible concern of a theory to a discipline, that is, 'how many of the basic problems in nursing or any of its specialities could be addressed by the same theory?' (Meleis 1991, 228). According to Walker and Avant (1995, 5), grand nursing theories are 'global conceptual frameworks defining broad perspectives for practice and ways of looking at nursing phenomena based on these perspectives'. What this means is that grand nursing theories tend to be concerned with the issues that have relevance for all of nursing. Not all grand nursing theories are at the same level of abstraction or have the same scope, but their general goal is to elucidate a world view, which is useful in understanding concepts and principles from a nursing perspective (Walker & Avant, 1995).

There was a proliferation of grand nursing theories in America in the 1960s and 1970s. For a detailed historical discussion, the reader is referred to McKenna (1997) and Meleis (1997). Since then, we would suggest, there has been a process akin to theoretical maturation occurring. While fewer grand theories were developed in the 1980s, nursing theorists have increasingly been revisiting, revising and refining their original theories with a view to developing them further. Although a similar proliferation of published grand theories has not been in evidence within the UK, there was an increase in activity in the 1990s. The best known grand theory in the UK is that of Roper et al (1996), although McKenna (1997) cites several others such as Castledine's (1986) stress adaptation model.

Some of these grand nursing theories were developed inductively from the theorist's experience in practice, while others were developed deductively from theories borrowed from other disciplines or developed by the theorists themselves. Others are a combination of both induction and deduction (see Ch. 1 for a discussion of induction and deduction).

Loosely speaking, grand nursing theories are a product of their time. Whether developed inductively or deductively, or both, all theories are value laden and are a product of the philosophical bent of the theorist as well as of the era in which the theorist was developing their work. For example, Peplau's (1952) theory was significantly influenced by Harry Stack Sullivan's theory of interpersonal relations (deductive) as well as by her extensive clinical experience working with psychiatric patients (inductive).

Similarly, when King (1971) began developing her work, she acknowledged that it had been heavily influenced by von Bertalanffy's (1956, 1968) general system theory; Orem (1971) recognised the influence of developmental theory, and Roy (1971) that of adaptation and general system theory. In the UK, Roper et al (1980) acknowledged the work of Henderson (1966) and the influence of Maslow's (1954) hierarchy of needs. However, all of these theorists have also made claims to inductive development arising out of their various clinical experiences, practice or research.

To some extent, these theories have been criticised for their mechanistic and possibly reductionist view of the person (see Ch. 1) (Benner & Wrubel 1989, Moody 1990), although the theorists themselves may reject this contention. While there may be some evidence that this is the case, it must be remembered that the dominant paradigm at the time of their development was that of the traditional sciences and the medical model was a pervasive influence in the nursing world. Hence their credibility and value in the outside scientific world would be judged against the rules and methods of this paradigm.

To illustrate this point further, Parse (1981) developed her theory in a period when the influence of the existentialists such as Merleau-Ponty and phenomenologists such as Heidegger was evident. Thus, her view of the person is one of 'the whole of the body and the person comprise the same entity' (Edwards 2001, 79; see 'Ontology' section in Ch. 1).

The current tendency to revisit, revise and refine grand nursing theories is in recognition that they are limited as they presently exist. Walker and Avant (1995) suggest that, although these theories have provided global perspectives for education, practice and administration, their generality and level of abstraction preclude testing. This inability to test the theories, as referred to earlier, will ultimately impact on their usefulness for the reality of practice.

Many readers will relate to this claim as they may have experienced attempts to use or apply one grand nursing theory to the practice setting. In previous decades there was some evidence of a blind acceptance of these theories without any attempt to evaluate their usefulness. When practitioners found anomalies in the application, they tended to become disillusioned and rejected these theories as having no relevance. However, the point is made here that they should never have been applied without evaluation. Grand nursing theories are largely concerned with nursing as it 'ought to be' rather than 'as it is'. There is a certain merit in this, if they are to change or influence nursing practice, but the manner in which they are introduced or adopted is significant if they are to continue to have any impact. We will return to this point when considering middle range theory.

Activity 3.4

Consider the model of nursing or model of care that you use in your practice setting. Think about the ways in which the model or framework is useful for your practice. Do you consider there are any ways in which its usefulness could be enhanced?

As previously mentioned, the concepts within grand nursing theories are highly abstract. Many of these theories, although not all, address the four metaparadigm concepts of person, health, environment and nursing. Fawcett (2000) claims this is an indication of a broad consensus within nursing as to its central concepts. However, the manner in which each theorist illuminates these concepts varies. The theorist makes a claim to a certain philosophical stance and indicates whether knowledge from another discipline has influenced the grand theory. This, in turn, impacts on how the concepts are presented. An important point here is that there should be congruence between the philosophical and knowledge claims, and the manner in which the concepts are delineated (Fawcett 2000).

The manner in which the metaparadigm concepts are presented, as well as the philosophical and knowledge claims, determines how such a grand nursing theory will be classified. Metatheorists such as Fawcett (2000), Marriner-Tomey (1998), Meleis (1997) and Stevens-Barnum (1998) all use categories to classify grand theories. McKenna (1997) claims this reflects other sciences that categorise those elements that are central to their discipline, such as botanists classifying plants, chemists classifying gases and biologists classifying cells.

In nursing, however, the classification systems are not agreed and metatheorists tend to present their own conception, which, of course, is another area where there is potential for confusion for the learner theorist. In addition, and to add to the complexity, there appear to be two levels of classification. The first is related to the paradigm or world view, and the second is concerned with broad categories of knowledge.

You may ask why the theorist's world view would be of concern to you in your practice. Simply stated, if you were considering adopting a grand nursing theory in your practice area, it should be congruent with the philosophical beliefs and values of that area. You would need to examine how the theorist presents the metaparadigm concepts in order to establish that congruence. For example, if you work in an emergency care setting, a theory such as Peplau's (1952), which is an interpersonal relationship theory, may not be appropriate. Alternatively, if you wanted to undertake a piece of research using a grand theory as a framework, you would need to be assured that the method you chose was congruent with its world view.

The least complex classification is that presented by Parse (1987), who classifies them as 'totality' and 'simultaneity' paradigms. To briefly demonstrate the differences between these paradigms using the four metaparadigm concepts, see below.

Totality

Person

- Organism that is composed of biopsychosocial and spiritual dimensions.

Environment

• The environment comprises internal and external stimuli.
• The person interacts with their environment and manipulates it to maintain health, life and so on.

Health

• Health is a dynamic state and is achieved when there is integrity and balance in the system.

Nursing

• Nursing practice is guided by a process where the patient's problems are assessed, a plan of care is drawn up, nursing actions or interventions are undertaken and outcomes are evaluated.
• Nursing care is directed towards persons who are deemed to be ill by society.
• Goals focus on care and cure of the sick, prevention of illness and health promotion.

Theorists that have been classified within this paradigm include King (1981), Orem (1995, 2001) and Roy and Andrews (1999), although they may not agree with it as it represents the mechanistic and reductionist view referred to earlier.

Simultaneity

Person

• Unitary being who is more than and different from the sum of their parts. The persons give meaning to their own situations and are responsible for choices they make in terms of moving beyond what currently exists.

Environment

• There is a continuous, mutual and simultaneous interaction between the person and their environment. To a large degree in this world view the person and their environment are one or inseparable.

Health

• Health is defined by the person. Health is concerned with the person's own perception of it and is related to perceived quality of life. Health consists of value priorities, that is, the person defines their own priorities and values as to what constitutes health for them. A definition of health is not possible, as health is defined by the person experiencing it.

Nursing

• Nursing practice is guided by the person who is receiving nursing care.
• Goals focus on quality of life but that which is determined by the person, not the nurse.
• The role of the nurse is to guide the way as determined by the person and care plans are not constructed around health problems.
• Given the view of health, society's view of illness is not significant in this world view.

Work that has been classified within this paradigm includes Newman (1994), Parse (1987) and Rogers (1970). Parse (1987) claims the totality paradigm remains dominant in nursing. To a certain degree it is not difficult to see why this is so. Many practising nurses will relate to or hold with the views proclaimed within the totality paradigm. Conversely, those of the simultaneity paradigm may challenge, in particular, our conceptions of health, and the role and goals of nursing. However, McKenna (1997) argues the simultaneity paradigm is gaining ground, particularly as a guide for research, education and theory. This is explained, partly, by the fact that the totality paradigm gives rise to research that is quantitative in nature, a tradition from which nursing has tried to disassociate itself. In contrast, the simultaneity paradigm accommodates research that is qualitative in nature, which, in the view of many nurses, is more appropriate in a human science such as nursing.

The second level of classification concerning categories of knowledge is also not generally agreed. However, the function of this classification also concerns congruence. As stated earlier, many of the current grand nursing theories were influenced by knowledge and theories from other disciplines. Fawcett (2000) has identified these as her classification system and they include:

• Systems
• Developmental
• Interaction

When a theorist acknowledges such an influence, it is important that the practitioner considering the grand nursing theory evaluates the claim. Each of the above three categories have certain characteristics, which you would then expect to see in the description of the four metaparadigm concepts of the grand nursing theory in question.

Furthermore, the classification would have some influence on your decision to adopt the framework. For example, Fawcett (2000) classifies some of the grand nursing theories thus:

Grand nursing theory	Category
King	Systems
Orem	Developmental
Roy	Systems with some characteristics of interaction

Having examined the characteristics of the category of knowledge and compared them to those in the grand nursing theory, you would then assess whether they were congruent with the beliefs and values of your practice area. For example, although Roy is classified as systems, she acknowledged the influence of adaptation theory and her model has been adopted in practice areas such as rehabilitation units where adaptation is considered the goal.

The final point in this section on grand nursing theories involves a return to the level of abstractness of the concepts within them. As previously stated, these theories are limited as they currently exist and, in recognition of this, theorists are now beginning to work on refinement and development. Part of this development is concerned with developing middle range theories from grand theories. In addition, Lenz et al (1995) claim the disciplines defining grand theories have achieved their role in legitimising the nursing discipline and, therefore, a shift to middle range theories is advocated. Middle range theories have shown a considerable growth in number in recent years.

MIDDLE RANGE THEORY

Walker and Avant's (1995) claim that, given the inherent difficulties associated with testing grand theories, a more workable level of theory was necessary, and these are known as middle range theories. They are formed of fewer concepts and are more limited in scope than grand theories. According to Lenz et al (1995, 1), they are abstract enough to extend beyond a given place, time or population, but specific enough and sufficiently close to empirical data to permit testing and to generate distinct questions for study or specific interventions for practice. Furthermore, developing and using middle range theories to underpin nursing research and practice are a promising approach to strengthening theory–research and theory–practice links.

McKenna (1997) identifies the risk of fragmentation of nursing's knowledge base, if middle range theory arbitrarily develops in all directions. Here is the value of identifying the phenomenon of interest to nursing, the importance of the metaparadigm and the place of grand theories that identify the boundaries of our interests. Thus, middle range theory is structured and, to a certain degree, the parameters for its development set in a broader context. Merton (1968, 39) has defined middle range theories as those

> that lie between the minor but necessary working hypotheses that evolve in abundance during day to day research and the all inclusive systematic efforts to develop unified theory that will explain all the observed uniformities of social behaviour, social organization and social change.

Liehr and Smith (1999) considered the requirements for classifying a theory as middle range. Using Chinn and Kramer's (1999) definition of theory, they proposed that key components, regardless of level of abstraction, were that the middle range theory presents its concepts and the definitions of those concepts. There is also an expectation that the structure of the theory is presented and the relationship between the concepts explicated. It is also seen as beneficial to include the approach for theory generation.

Their criteria reflect general clarity and consistency in determining what can be defined as middle range theory. However, as with grand theories, there is some variation in scope and level of abstraction within the range of what are seen as middle range theories. This variation had led Lenz (1996) (cited in Liehr & Smith 1999) to suggest there may be some benefit in recognising levels of theory within the overall middle range theory level. Liehr and Smith (1999) propose three categories of abstraction in their survey.

Levels of abstraction	Example
High middle	caring
Middle	chronic sorrow
Low middle	acute pain management

Lenz (1996) (cited in Liehr & Smith 1999) has identified some approaches for middle range theory development and these include:

- inductive theory building through research and practice
- deductive theory building from grand nursing theories
- combining existing nursing and non-nursing theories
- deriving theories from other disciplines
- synthesising theories from published research findings
- developing theories from clinical practice guidelines (Liehr and Smith (1999) expand this to include practice guidelines and standards rooted in research).

Liehr and Smith (1999), in their article surveying middle range theories in nursing, found evidence that all of the above approaches, except that of synthesising theory from published research, had been used. Although the above list is by no means prescriptive or definitive, it gives some indication of the range of possible methods that can fruitfully be adopted when developing middle range theory.

McKenna (1997) claims middle range theories are often developed inductively using qualitative research methods—a view supported by Liehr and Smith (1999). An example of a middle range theory developed in this way is Eakes et al's (1998) middle range theory of chronic sorrow. The theory was developed using concept analysis, a critical review of the research and validation of ten qualitative studies of various loss situations.

Good and Moore (1996) inductively developed a middle range theory of acute pain from clinical practice guidelines. Good (1998) developed this work further by deducing testable hypotheses and extending the original theory.

Deductive theory building from grand theories has been undertaken by the original theorists, such as King (1981) and Orem (1995). Orem has derived three middle range theories from her conceptual model (grand theory) self care framework. They are the theory of self care, theory of nursing system and the theory of self care deficit. King (1981) derived her theory of goal attainment from her general systems framework. These initiatives are examples of how grand nursing theories can be developed and subsequently validated or even not validated. The use of grand theories as a framework for developing middle range theories has not been confined to the original theorists. For example, Olson and Hanchett (1997) developed a middle range theory of nurse expressed empathy and patient distress from Orlando's (1961) theory.

In addition, middle range theory development has not been restricted to derivation from grand nursing theories. For instance, Reed (1991) developed a middle range theory of self transcendence from developmental theory and Auvil-Novak (1997), in developing a theory of chronotherapeutic intervention for post-surgical pain, generated it from chronobiologic theory.

The relationship with and implications for practice of middle range theories can be highlighted using Auvil-Novak's (1997) theory as an example. Having validated her theory in three research studies, the findings suggested that analgesic effectiveness and analgesic requirements of patients post-operatively had a temporal (time) variation. More or less analgesia was required depending on the time of the day. The theory proposes that analgesic therapy that is delivered in harmony with the individual's pain rhythm will enhance the post-operative outcome for the patient. She also suggested that the PCA (patient-controlled analgesia) pump provides a method for identifying individual pain rhythms and assessing individual pain and could be readily used by nurses in the clinical practice setting.

At present, the bulk of the published work on middle range theories appears to originate, as with grand nursing theories, in America. It is suggested that, within the UK setting, this may reflect the earlier reluctance in

America to label work at this level theory. However, it is proposed that, with increasing theoretical confidence, middle range theory development will receive increasing attention.

Activity 3.5

Using some of the examples of middle range theory outlined in this section as a
  guide, think of an area of your practice that is based on a middle range theory. It
  could be derived/adapted/adopted from another discipline or one that is unique to
  nursing.
Now outline how it impacts on your practice.
How do you think it might be developed further?

PRACTICE THEORY

According to Walker and Avant (1995), one result of metatheory is the emergence of the notion of practice theory. Jacox (1974, 10) defined practice theory as 'theory that says given this nursing goal (producing some desired change or effect in the patient's condition), these are the actions the nurse must take to meet the goal (produce the change)'.

For instance, a nursing goal may be to prevent a patient developing a pressure ulcer. Nursing practice states that one of the actions that must be taken to prevent pressure ulcers is to relieve pressure. Thus, the nurse instigates a programme of pressure relief. Therefore, as Walker and Avant (1995, 12) state, 'the essence of practice theory is a desired goal and prescription for action to meet that goal'.

Activity 3.6

In order to situate practice theory, consider the example above related to the prevention
  of pressure ulcers.
How do you know about the existence of pressure ulcers?
How do you know one of the actions to prevent pressure ulcers is to relieve pressure?
How do you know what the programme of pressure relief should involve?

If you consider your answers to these questions, practice theory presupposes the existence of other levels of theory. Dickoff and James (1968) and Dickoff et al (1968) propose there are four levels of theory, the highest level of which is situation-producing or practice theory. They also maintain that theory at this highest level cannot be generated until theory at the preceding levels has been devised. They name the levels that roughly correspond to describing, explaining, predicting and controlling (Walker & Avant 1995) as:

First level—naming or factor-isolating theories
Second level—factor-relating theories
Third level—situation-relating theories that incorporate:

  –predictive theories
  –promoting or inhibiting theories.
Fourth level—situation-producing theories (prescriptive or practice
  theories)

A brief outline of the first three levels is presented here in order to put into context fourth-level theory, which is discussed in more detail. First-level or naming theory is concerned with naming, describing and classifying concepts. In terms of names that are less than informative, perhaps an abstract concept, Dickoff et al (1968) propose that a function of factor-isolating theory is to name the elements of that concept. To have theories at this level, they claim, is to have a terminology. This level of theory development constitutes descriptive theory (Meleis 1991, 1997). For example, pressure ulcer is a concept that succinctly describes the phenomenon whereby an ulcer results from pressure. We know, however, that in the past these were also described as bed sores, decubitus ulcers and pressure sores. If we examine the term 'bed sores', it does not adequately convey the properties of the phenomenon. However, while pressure ulcer conveys some characteristics of the phenomenon, we know that pressure-ulcer grading systems have been developed in order to clarify the term 'pressure ulcer'. Similarly, in naming the characteristics of pressure, we would be concerned with what type of pressure, how low/high the pressure is and so on.

Second-level or factor-relating theory is the next level of complexity, and it concerns seeing things in relation to each other. These statements describe or depict the relationship between the named concepts. Meleis (1991, 1997) describes these as descriptive theories of the explanatory kind. For instance, we would state the relationship between the two named concepts of pressure and pressure ulcer. This could simply be stating there is a relationship or could tentatively predict the relationship.

Third-level or situation-relating theories are more widely known as predictive theories and are predicting theories. Simply stated, these theories make a prediction about the relationship between the concepts. Dickoff et al (1968) note that this level of theorising also incorporates promoting or inhibiting theories. This is simply demonstrated as follows:

- Prediction: X causes Y to happen. Pressure causes pressure ulcers.
- Promoting: What causes Y to follow X more quickly or promotes it?
  Increased/unrelieved pressure increases the incidence of pressure ulcers.
- Inhibiting: What causes Y to follow X more slowly or inhibit it?
  Reducing/relieving pressure reduces the incidence of pressure ulcers.

According to Meleis' (1991, 1997) classification, fourth-level theory is prescriptive theory. The previous three levels of theory are precursors for situation-producing or fourth-level theory. That is, if the concepts have been named, the relationships between them established and predictions between relationships delineated, situation-producing theory considers how desired situations can be brought about. Put more simply, we know from third-level theory that X *causes Y to happen* or, in our example, *reducing X reduces the incidence of Y.*

If we assume that Y is a desirable condition or outcome, fourth-level or situation-producing theory is about *enabling X to happen or come about* or *facilitating X so that Y can happen.*

Dickoff et al (1968, 421) outline the three essential ingredients of situation-producing theory:

- Goal content specified as the aim for activity.
- Prescriptions for activity to realise the goal content.
- A survey list to serve as a supplement to the prescriptions for activity and as preparation for future prescription for activity towards the goal content.

The first essential ingredient of situation-producing theory is the conceptualisation of a goal content. In determining the goal content, there should be some specific reference to the value of the goal content as being something that is desirable. *For example, the patient will be free from pressure ulcers.*

The second ingredient of prescriptions for activity is concerned with that activity that will bring about the goal. The prescription for activity gives a directive regarding an agent or agents with a specific end in mind. An important point is that this activity takes place in a 'particular' situation. *For example, the list of activities that would need to be undertaken in order to prevent pressure ulcers.*

The third essential ingredient, the survey list, concerns two aspects. Firstly, those factors or aspects of the activity that are relevant to the situation but which may not be at the level of a prescription or directive and, secondly, other theories that may be relevant to the situation and should be taken into account in order to enhance the possibility of achieving the desired situation.

In addition to these factors, the survey list includes the particulars of a given situation. This is where Dickoff et al (1968) include the 'judgement', of, say, the nurse in this case, about the particular patient at a given time and in a given place. This they claim involves judging the salient features of a particular situation and making adjustments to routine activity in the light of anything specific.

Dickoff et al (1968) consider there are six aspects of activity in the survey list that correspond with six questions about the activity. Using our pressure ulcer example, these are as follows:

1. Agency—who or what performs the activity?
   – The level of skills required by the nurse including experience, knowledge, practical skills.

–Theories regarding agency that may be deemed relevant.
In managing the prevention of pressure ulcers, for example, who will undertake the risk assessment? What skills are needed in order to do so? Who will implement the actions? Is it acceptable to have an unqualified nurse undertake these activities?

2. Patiency or recipiency—who or what is the recipient of the activity?
   –Characteristics of the recipient (patient).
   –Relevant theories about the recipient that may influence the situation, for example, age, condition, cultural issues.

For example, how will the healing process be affected by the age of the patient receiving care for prevention of pressure ulcers?

3. Framework—in what context is the activity performed?
   –Environmental or other contextual issues that may influence the performance of the activities or influence the goal content or outcome.
   –Theories about contextual issues that inform the activity.

For example, if the patient had spinal surgery, how will that impact on the equipment to be used in the prevention of pressure ulcers?

4. Terminus—what is the end point of the activity?
   –Identifying the end point or knowing when the end point has been achieved—how and when is evaluation undertaken?
   –Theories about achievement of outcome that may be relevant.

What is accomplished by the activity of preventing pressure ulcers? How do we know when the risk has passed or has changed?

5. Procedure—what is the guiding procedure, technique or protocol of the activity?
   –Are there any clinical guidelines or protocols that support the proposed activity?
   –Theories that underpin the guidelines or protocols that may be relevant.

How often do we move the patient? How do we know how often to do it? How will knowing about pressure and capillary pressure in particular help us?

6. Dynamics—what is the energy source for the activity: whether chemical, physical, biological, mechanical or psychological?
   –How is the activity going to be performed, that is, what source of energy will be used—is it a mechanical activity, for example, moving and handling?
   –Theories that are relevant regarding the energy source, such as ergonomics.

How do we use the mechanical hoist? Is it suitable for this patient? How is the hoist to be used? How will the patient's psychological state impact on the prescribed actions for the prevention of pressure ulcers?

Given the focus on practice in Dickoff et al's (1968) proposal for theory in nursing at a situation-producing level, it is not surprising that it generated considerable debate among nurses who were proposing unique theory for nursing. Furthermore, the notion of practice theory legitimises both nursing practice and the existence of nursing theory. However, it has also been questioned from a number of perspectives.

Walker and Avant (1995) claim that, if practice theory were separated from its base in predictive (third level) theory, the use of the word theory is generous. They argue that nurses may wish to drop the word 'theory' and think of practice theory as 'nursing practices'. It is countered here in that Dickoff et al (1968) clearly state that the preceding levels of theory exist for the next one in the hierarchy and using their model or framework necessitates maintaining the relationship with predictive (third-level) theory.

McKenna (1997) makes the case that, as fourth-level theory is aimed at prescription (control), then it is heavily influenced by the traditional or positivist view of science. He supports his argument by highlighting that the hierarchical nature of the four levels of theory means that fourth-level is better than first-level theory for nursing. He goes on to say that, if practice theory is based on cause and effect, then experimental research designs are those that nurses would have to use. This position is countered by the argument that Dickoff et al's (1968) framework allows for plurality of research designs in describing, explaining, predicting and prescribing (controlling) phenomena of interest to nursing. The central issue is one of purpose, and naming theory has ultimately the same end purpose as situation-producing theory, that is, practice.

A further point in relation to Dickoff et al's (1968) framework is the notion of 'judgement' in the survey list. They see judgement as experience, practical wisdom or practical insight. They go on to say an important feature of judgement is 'the capacity—usually with the smooth directness of habit and the lightening speed that makes us think of insight as deep rather than broad—to consult all salient features in a particular situation . . . ' (p. 422). Thus, it is proposed here that their framework accommodates what Benner (1984) refers to as 'know how' or practical knowledge (see Ch. 2). To a certain degree, it also corresponds with Schön's (1983) reflection-in-action, where problems are solved for practice through informal theories that are being constantly tested, modified and retested in 'on-the-spot' experimenting (Rolfe 1997, 94) (see Ch. 9 on reflection). In the survey list, then, the relationship between 'formal' theory and 'informal' theory is established where the practitioner's knowledge of formal theory will form part of the process of making a judgement about a particular situation but where some modification for the given situation might be appropriate. For example, a practitioner may have knowledge of a bereavement or grief model, and will use that knowledge when responding to a person who is grieving. However, in the given situation with a particular person, the practitioner may adjust their response in recognition of issues or variables that are pertinent to that individual or situation.

Beckstrand (1980) takes issue with the notion that nursing is concerned with practice theory. She claims that for practice theory to exist it should be different to scientific and ethical knowledge, which she argues are all that constitute the knowledge base of nursing. Others who argue that nursing does not need its own theory posit that nursing can use theory borrowed from other disciplines as the basis for describing, explaining and predicting the phenomena of interest (Meleis 1997). The use of borrowed theories in nursing has received some attention. Meleis (1991) claims that there is an element in nursing where that which is 'imported' is superior to that which is developed by nurses themselves. However, in the early stages of theo-retical development in nursing, theories were taken from other disciplines and used in nursing practice. Some of these theories were adopted within nursing without any adaptation, theories of classical conditioning being an example, claims McKenna (1997). Others were taken and adapted to the sit-uation in which they were to be applied. Timpson (1996, 1031) claims that, once borrowed theories have been transmuted to a nursing context, then they constitute nursing theory because they comprise shared knowledge employed in a distinctive way.

Finally, having delineated the four levels of theory in nursing, Walker and Avant (1995) clarify the relationship between each level when they state that metatheory clarifies grand level theory through explication of the broad interests of the discipline. Grand-level theory guides the develop-ment of middle range theory, which in turn directs practice theory. Practice-level theory tests middle range theory, which refines grand-level theory and ultimately provides material for metatheory level.

SUMMARY

This chapter has considered the world of theory. The initial focus of the chapter was an exploration of some of the characteristics of theory. It was outlined that theories concerned some aspects of the world and were often grouped in terms of their interest for a particular discipline. It was noted that theory does not necessarily describe reality, but speculates on what it might be or what it ought to be. Other characteristics that were considered included phenomena, concepts and propositions.

Two definitions of theory were offered to demonstrate how differing world views impact on whether a conception is regarded as theory.

Whether nursing theory exists or not was discussed, taking into consideration the definitions outlined.

Walker and Avant's (1995) framework for levels of theory was used to explore metatheory, grand-level theory, middle range theory and practice theory. Metatheory focused on the issues of general concern to nursing particularly, and some exploration of the role of metatheorists was undertaken. Grand-level theory was considered with particular reference to conceptual frameworks and/or models of nursing. Middle range theory was outlined with reference to some of the work that is currently being undertaken and the new focus in the discipline towards developing this level of theory. Finally, practice theory was examined with consideration of Dickoff and James (1968) and Dickoff et al's (1968) four levels of theory.

The final question for this chapter concerns where we (nursing) go from here. There appears to be a drive towards developing middle range theory that has relevance for practice and it is anticipated that this will gain momentum in the twenty-first century. This will not only enable grand-level theory to be evaluated in terms of its relevance for the practice of nursing, but will enable consolidation of the relationship between middle range and practice theory. Liehr and Smith (1999) believe nursing theory will move forward through the creation of middle range theory and this movement will give substance and direction to the discipline.

4

What is the relationship between nursing theory, research and practice?

INTRODUCTION

This chapter is concerned with examining the relationship between theory, research and practice, with a particular focus on the theory research links. As stated at the beginning of the last chapter, theory provides knowledge about the world. Its value is that it structures, and provides direction for and organization of knowledge deemed to be important to a discipline. However, as Dickoff et al (1968) claim, in order for theory to be useful, it must be determined whether it fits reality. In a practice-based discipline such as nursing, reality is clinical practice and reality is consulted through research. In other words, theory provides knowledge about the world of clinical practice through research.

It is this relationship that is the focus of this chapter. The interdependency between theory, research and practice will be explored. This will include a brief insight into the nature of research. Links between theory and research will be examined using Chinn and Kramer's (1999) structure of theory generation and theory validation. However, other classifications of the relationship will also be presented to widen the discussion. These are particularly useful in highlighting the range of research methods that can be employed to generate or test all levels of theory at all stages of development. Implicit and explicit reference to clinical practice will be undertaken throughout.

INTENDED LEARNING OUTCOMES

By the end of this chapter you will:

1. have an understanding of the relationship between theory, research and practice

2. have some insight into research in nursing
3. be able to articulate the nature of the links between theory and research
4. be able to differentiate between theory generation and theory validation
5. have some insight into one model for the development of theory.

Activity 4.1
Before we progress to discuss what is the relationship between theory, research and practice, consider what you think it might be.

THEORY, RESEARCH AND PRACTICE

According to McKenna (1997, 221) 'there are three core elements in any practice discipline—research, theory and practice', a claim that appears to find general agreement in the literature. Meleis (1997) states that the nature of nursing science and its potential for growth necessitates a close relationship between theory, research and practice, if the ultimate objective of understanding, enhancing, promoting and facilitating the health care needs of clients and communities is to be achieved.

Dickoff et al (1968, 415) assert that this relationship between nursing theory, nursing practice and nursing research is mutually interrelated and interdependent (see Fig. 4.1). They go on to claim that

theory is born in practice, is refined in research and must and can return to practice if research is to be other than a draining off of energy from the main business of nursing and theory more than idle speculation.

Research, according to Pryjmachuk (1996) forms the link between theory and practice, and he believes it to be the key to the development of a

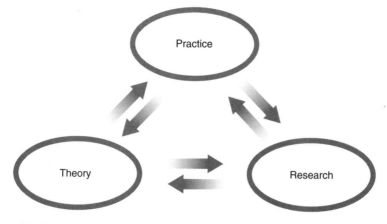

Figure 4.1   Relationship between theory, research and practice.

discipline. Fealy (1997) contends that the relationship between theory and practice operates in both directions, where theory helps determine practice but practice is itself essential in the development of theoretical concepts in nursing.

Yet Pryjmachuk (1996) argues that many nurses lack a true understanding of the interrelationship between the three concepts. To a certain degree, this can be explained by the traditional view of the relationship between theory and practice. This is reflected in Walker's (1992) argument that theory and practice are distinct and separate endeavours, where pre-eminence is given to theory. Theory is seen as objective evidence derived from research investigations, the results of which are used to guide and regulate practice. Fealy (1997) states this view of the theory–practice relationship has its basis in the natural science view. The prominence of this position, argues Rolfe (1998) is reflected in calls for all practice to be based on research or evidence. He goes on to claim that this creates a hierarchical relationship between theoreticians and practitioners, and between theory and practice, where research generates knowledge that builds, supports or tests theory and, most significantly, dictates to or determines practice. As a result of this view, Meleis (1997) asserts that nursing practice, as a significant area for theory development, has been neglected for many decades.

While Walker's position is waning in contemporary nursing, its influence has been pervasive in terms of how practitioners view theory and research. Levine (1995, 11) suggested that attempts to 'justify theory by forcing its use in contexts where it barely fits have contributed to the increasing disenchantment' with it. It could be argued that, for many, theory has become a side issue removed from everyday nursing practice.

A further issue concerning the relationship between theory, research and practice is the argument as to whether research must always be related to theory, that is either isolated or theory-linked research. According to Chinn and Kramer (1999), theory-linked research is designed to develop, refine or test theory. Conversely, isolated research is not linked to the processes of theory development and is more limited in terms of what it can contribute to the discipline even though it may be of excellent quality. However, Dickoff and James (1968) and Meleis (1997) believe that research that is not done in the context of theory is pointless and theory that is produced without research has little hope of being viable. For example, an isolated research study or project may be undertaken, but the findings may not be reported. Thus, the process is incomplete and the potential for contribution to the development of theory is lost (Meleis 1997).

In order to understand Dickoff and James' (1968) and Meleis' (1997) claims, we must refer back to the broadly encompassing view of what constitutes theory explored in Chapter 3. If we accept that theory can range from primitive to sophisticated or well developed, then there is the potential for all research to be theory linked in some way. For example, Meleis

(1997) claims that, if we have a 'hunch' about the relationship between concepts, then we have begun the process of theory development.

To illustrate this claim, let us return to first-level or 'naming' theory (see Ch. 3). We observe, in practice, that the word 'trust' is commonly used in reference to the relationship between the nurse and the patient. We also observe, however, that there appear to be differences in how each practitioner views trust and this seems to impact on how the nurse–patient relationship is conceived. This sense of disquiet might lead us to consider undertaking a concept analysis of trust with the initial aim of achieving consistency in how the term is viewed. This is part of theorising, if we subscribe to Dickoff and James' (1968) definition of theory and is labelled stimulating production of theory. They maintain there are eight kinds of research that encompass either stimulating production of the theory or testing the theory at each of the four levels they believe exist.

Others, such as Rolfe (1998), believe there is a difference between what he refers to as theoretical research and clinical research, where the former is concerned with generating and testing theory, and the latter with improving the care and treatment of individual patients. However, his view of theoretical research appears to indicate an interpretation of theory that is more in line with that of McKay (1969) (see Ch. 3) than that of Dickoff and James (1968) and Meleis (1997). He associates theoretical research with generalisable laws and principles, and does not appear to accept that theory can exist at various levels, or can and must be born in practice.

Disenchantment with research also appears to exist amongst practitioners who see it as a highly specialised and possibly elitist activity. This, in some ways, has been affected by the incorporation of nursing into institutes of higher education and a feeling that research is removed from practice. The Department of Health (1995) state the 'doing' of research is not suited to every practitioner but that every practitioner should be involved in using the findings of research. The subsequent perception, therefore, is that research findings are passed 'down' to practitioners, who will then implement them.

However, Rolfe (1998) maintains that experienced nurses who may claim they base their practice on research findings are actually more likely to listen to their professional judgement than the research findings, that is, 'theories-in-use' as opposed to 'espoused' theories (see Ch. 9 for a discussion of these).

Yet the view that practice should be based on research is well documented and represented by Parahoo (1997, 4) who states 'practice without research is like building castles on slippery ground' and 'research without practice is like building castles in the air'. The contention is based on the assumption that practice that is not based on research must be based on tradition or intuition, and is, therefore, unsound (Rolfe 1998).

There are some difficulties with the notion of research-based practice in nursing. Primarily as an emerging discipline or one that is striving to establish its knowledge base, research findings may not exist to support all areas of practice. As was seen in the previous chapter, many of the theories in nursing are in development, and are still being generated, refined and tested by research. As Parahoo (1997) states, much remains to be achieved.

Secondly, Benner (1984) and others have suggested the knowledge embedded in clinical practice is an important source of expertise, as the clinician tests and refines propositions, hypotheses and principle-based expectations in actual practice situations. However, if the doing of research is a specialist activity, then practitioner-based research may not be seen as desirable or considered valuable. As a practice-based discipline, the question is can we afford to allow nursing practice as a source of theory and research to be further neglected because of an elitist position regarding the 'doing' of research? As Lindsay (1990, 35) claims 'each nurse needs to recognise that the theorist, researcher and practitioner exist to some extent in all of us'. Therefore, as with theory, a broad conception of what constitutes research is necessary.

Activity 4.2

When you consider the word 'research', what does it mean to you?

RESEARCH

What do we mean when we say it is necessary to have a broad conception of research? The word 'research' is derived from the Old French *recercher* meaning to 'seek' (*Chambers English Dictionary* 1995). Its contemporary meaning is generally associated with the notion of enquiry. Therefore, research is a tool of science, not an activity for its own sake, whose function is enquiry (Dickoff & James 1968). According to Burns and Groves (2001, 3), research is 'diligent, systematic inquiry or investigation to validate and refine existing knowledge and generate new knowledge'. However, within this broad definition, there are disagreements as to what constitutes diligent and systematic inquiry.

In order to explain this, let us return again to Kuhn's notion of paradigms as discussed in Chapter 1. If you recall, members of a scientific community subscribe to a paradigm, and accept its laws and rules about the focus of its work, the way problems are approached and resolved, and the manner in which its research is conducted. Nursing, in its early efforts to develop its knowledge base and move to professional status, subscribed to the rules and methods of the traditional sciences and medicine. The 'gold standard' research method was, and perhaps still is, the experimental method, and the randomised controlled trial (RCT) (Hicks 1998) in particular, under the umbrella of quantitative research. Control, randomisation, objectivity of the researcher, measurement through statistical analysis and generalisability are key features, where the overall aim is to eliminate bias and erroneous conclusions. The pressure on nursing to operate as a large-scale science (Meerabeau 1997) by adhering to these rules results in efforts to measure the phenomena of interest and achieve generalisation about human conditions. Such is its influence that often those who manage funding applications for research studies look at it through a randomised clinical trial lens and applications using alternative types of evidence are often rejected as anecdotal or subjective (Hicks 1998, Meerabeau 1997). Furthermore, Hicks (1998) claims the RCT is almost the unquestioned method in the drive for evidence-based health care.

Rolfe (1998) counters this by claiming that it is not possible to take the findings from these types of studies and apply them to individual patients, communities or contexts. He offers the example of predictors of suicide risk. Studies have indicated there is a statistical correlation between suicide and the elderly, suicide and young men, and suicide and employment. While such information is useful, it does not enable a practitioner in a particular context with a particular patient to make an accurate prediction as to the likelihood of that person committing suicide (Rolfe 1998, 676).

This does not mean that findings resulting from studies using experimental methods should be rejected. What it does mean, however, is that there is a need for alternative approaches to address some of the phenomena of interest in nursing. These alternative approaches have largely been classified under the heading of qualitative research, although in recent years triangulation, that is, the use of multiple methods to study the same phenomena, has also been advocated. An example of triangulation and the most common type used is methodological, where two or more research methods or procedures are used in one study (Burns & Groves 2001).

In summary, then, research in nursing is broadly categorised as quantitative, qualitative and triangulation. However, Parahoo (1997) issues a caution when he states the assumption that quantitative research is associated with quantity, and qualitative research with description and quality is too simplistic and unhelpful. He believes that examining the underpinning philosophical assumptions, methods of data collection and data analysis is useful in distinguishing between quantitative and qualitative research studies. Table 4.1 outlines the general characteristics of qualitative and quantitative research. However, it is recommended that the reader consult a research textbook for more detailed discussion than that provided here.

In any study or project, the emergent research question or hypothesis plays a part in determining the choice of approach. However, for the purposes of the relationship between theory, research and practice, it is the process preceding the arrival at a research question or hypothesis that is important for this discussion. For example, did your question derive from observation of a phenomenon in practice? Is it a phenomenon that has not

Table 4.1   Characteristics of qualitative and quantitative research

Quantitative	Qualitative
The world is stable and predictable	The world is dynamic
Truth is found in common laws	Truth is found in changing patterns
Generalisation is highly valued	Uniqueness is highly valued
Elicits 'hard data'	Elicits 'soft data'
Seeking causal relationships	Concerned with discovery and description
Boundaries between researcher and subject are defined—objectivity is valued	There is integration between researcher and participant—interaction is valued
Variables controlled and effect observed	Explain variables—researcher immersed in the context
Strict sampling criteria to enable statistical testing—usually large numbers. Random selection and assignment of subjects	Sampling criteria bound to the phenomena under investigation—usually small numbers
Data collection—questionnaires (closed questions), highly structured interviews	Data collection—questionnaires (open), interviews (semistructured and unstructured), critical incident analysis, participant observation
Data analysis—statistical—use of standard measuring tools	Data analysis—comparative analysis, coding, categorising, patterning, identifying paradigm cases
Rigour—reliability and validity (internal and external)	Rigour—credibility, transferability (fittingness), dependability, fruitfulness

been named or is it one about which little is known? Alternatively, are you considering taking a known theory from nursing or another discipline, and considering how it would be applicable to your area of practice? Are you investigating a causal relationship between concepts in practice?

Several writers (Chinn & Kramer 1999, McKenna 1997, Meleis 1997) have constructed frameworks or outlined strategies for structuring this relationship (see Table 4.2). Each strategy proposes a relationship between research, practice and theory, and as the nature of the relationship differs, so too does the type of research undertaken.

There are similar characteristics across each model but, for simplicity, that proposed by Chinn and Kramer (1999) is used here. However, reference to the others will be made, where appropriate.

Table 4.2   Strategies for linking theory, research and practice

Meleis (1997)	McKenna (1997)	Chinn and Kramer (1999)
Theory practice theory	Theory testing	Theory generating
Practice theory	Theory generating	Theory validating
Research theory	Theory evaluating	
Theory research theory	Theory framing	
Integrated		

THEORY-GENERATING RESEARCH

In theory-generating research, theories are developed, usually, inductively (from the specific to the general—see Ch. 1). It is about generating and describing relationships without preconceived ideas of what the phenomenon might mean (Chinn & Kramer 1999). Although it is impossible, by virtue of being human and existing in the world, not to have preconceived ideas, in theory-generating research, the researcher must attempt to be as open as possible to the phenomenon under study.

Theory-generating research is often concerned with phenomena about which little is known. Therefore, the purpose is to explore these phenomena in the context or world in which they occur. The world of nursing practice provides a rich source for the study of such phenomena, which has been evidenced by the increasing interest in theory-generation research, for example middle range theories, as discussed in Chapter 3.

However, there are two distinct philosophical schools of thought which use induction as a means of generating theory. The result is that theory can be generated through both qualitative and quantitative research approaches.

When the researcher begins with practice, Meleis (1997) refers to it as practice theory strategy. The process commences with a nagging question or observation that arises in a practice situation. There is an assumption that existing theories do not provide the answer, yet the phenomenon is deemed important enough to pursue. It may be that some insight into the phenomenon already exists but has not been articulated. Subsequently, phenomena are labelled, concepts are developed, properties of the concepts are described and propositions developed (see Ch. 5 on concept analysis).

Activity 4.3

Think of an area of your practice about which you have a concern or a question. Describe what it is that concerns you about that aspect of practice.

Meleis (1997) declares this strategy is heavily based on the work of Glaser and Strauss (1967) and is widely known as grounded theory. It has its foundation in the social sciences and symbolic interactionism. Grounded theory involves a systematic set of procedures used to arrive at theory about the social processes in groups (Lo-Biondo-Wood & Haber 1998). Observation is emphasised and data collection, coding and categorisation occur simultaneously. Concepts are formed and relationships between them proposed. Grounded theory processes involve formulating, testing and redeveloping propositions until a theory emerges (Burns & Groves 2001).

Ethnography is another form of theory-generating research, originating in cultural anthropology, and was developed in order to accommodate the in-depth study of cultures through members of that culture. Culture, for the purposes of, say, using ethnography in nursing studies, is defined by commonalities within a social group. Therefore, studies might concentrate on a unit or subculture of the larger social grouping. For example, a researcher may wish to explore the subculture of patients who are experiencing a particular phenomenon, like diabetes or chronic heart disease. The researcher's goal is to understand the native's view of their own world. This is also known as the emic (insider's) view. The researcher enters the world of the participants to view what happens, listen to what the members of the culture say, ask questions and collect whatever data are available. The data should eventually lead to propositions about the culture/subculture under investigation (Lo-Biondo-Wood & Haber 1998).

Chinn and Kramer (1999) maintain that, as some phenomena cannot be observed directly, theory generating research must sometimes use indirect ways of gathering data. One such approach is that of phenomenology that is grounded in philosophy and whose focus is the explication of the individual's 'lived experience'. Phenomenology acknowledges and values the meanings people ascribe to their own existence (Taylor 1993). As these experiences and meanings cannot be directly observed, they can only be accessed through articulation by the person experiencing them. Phenomenology is complex and the reader is advised to read further on its tenets as the description here is limited.

Each of the above inductive approaches produces a different kind of knowledge (Chinn & Kramer 1999). Grounded theory methods result in propositions joining new or existing concepts together (Chinn & Kramer 1999, McKenna 1997). Ethnographic studies lead to new ways of viewing phenomena and phenomenology generally results in interpreted narrative that describes the meaning of an experience as fully as possible.

Activity 4.4

Referring back to the concern you identified in Activity 4.3, consider how any of the above research approaches might be useful in helping you to investigate your concern.

The above approaches are generally classed as qualitative, but inductive theory generation is also undertaken using quantitative approaches and is concomitant with Meleis' (1997) research theory strategy. Meleis (1997) claims this strategy is the most acknowledged and accepted by scientists in many fields including nursing. Those who subscribe to this view believe theory development occurs exclusively as a result of replicated and confirmed research. From this viewpoint, theories are signified as scientific theories. Their purpose is to put the knowledge of their respective fields together so that it is systematically organised into theories that describe, explain and predict a part of the world.

This strategy assumes that there is truth out there in real life that can be verified or refuted. The more a hypothesis is verified, the more it is assumed that this truth exists. This strategy also presumes that there is general agreement in the community of scientists regarding the major concepts of concern, and that the research projects or studies consider a manageable number of variables (Meleis 1997). In this process there are four steps, which include:

1. selecting a phenomenon and listing all its characteristics
2. measuring all the characteristics of the phenomenon in as many situations as possible
3. analysing the data to determine systematic patterns that may be worthy of further attention
4. having identified the patterns, organizing them into theoretical statements that form the 'laws of nature'
(Reynolds 1971).

From a quantitative research perspective, descriptive studies, correlational research, quasi-experimental and experimental research may be employed, depending on which step of the process the researcher is at. For example, descriptive research provides a precise account of the phenomena being studied and is a way of discovering new meaning, describing what already exists, identifying the frequency of an occurrence and/or categorising information (Burns & Groves 2001). The most commonly used descriptive research design is that of the descriptive/exploratory survey (Lo-Biondo-Wood & Haber 1998). The results of these studies will often provide the potential hypotheses to direct correlational, quasi-experimental or experimental studies.

Correlational research involves the examination of the relationship between two or more variables. It is not the purpose of these studies to determine cause and effect, but it is to quantify (measure) the strength of the relationship between the variables under study.

The purpose of quasi-experimental and experimental research is to examine the cause and effect relationship between variables. According to Burns and Groves (2001), there are very few 'pure' experimental studies in nursing and there is a tendency to take quasi-experimental approaches. In quasi-experimental studies, some aspect, such as the treatment variable, the sample or the context or setting of the study, has not been controlled or manipulated, usually because it cannot be. Thus, quasi-experimental studies are seen as less powerful (Burns & Groves 2001). Examples of quasi-experimental studies are those that attempt to determine the impact of nursing interventions on patient outcome. For example, does preoperative teaching regarding patient-controlled analgesia impact on the patient's pain behaviour postoperatively?

Activity 4.5

Referring back to the concern you identified in Activity 4.3, consider whether any of the above research approaches might be useful in helping you to investigate your concern.

According to McKenna (1997, 204), findings from theory generation research may lead to:

- the formulation of a new theory
- support for an existing theory
- rejection of an existing theory
- adaptation or revision of an existing theory.

The theories that emerge from theory-generation research can be either descriptive, explanatory or predictive/prescriptive theories (see Dickoff & James on levels of theory in Ch. 3). Generally, and as stated previously, the findings are stated in the form of concepts or propositions. The level of sophistication or the type of propositional statements indicates the level of theory being generated.

If you recall in Chapter 3, we referred to propositions as being features of theories, and noted that Fawcett and Downs (1992) differentiated them into relational and nonrelational, as does Meleis (1997). Nonrelational propositions are concerned with one concept only, therefore, the theory generated is descriptive. Fawcett and Downs (1992), McKenna (1997), Meleis (1997) and Walker and Avant (1995) have proposed types of nonrelational proposition that are represented diagrammatically in Table 4.3.

Nonrelational propositions could be said to be precursors of relational propositions. As Walker and Avant (1995) state, attempts to describe, explain or predict phenomena must start with a clear understanding of what is to be described, explained or predicted. For example, if there are few or no concepts available in the area of interest, then nonrelational propositions can be developed through concept derivation or concept synthesis. Concept derivation describes the process of taking a concept from

Table 4.3 Nonrelational propositions (concerned with one concept only)

Proposition type	Definition
Existence propositions	Describes and asserts the existence of one concept
Definitional propositions comprising:	Describes the characteristics of a concept
Theoretical	Dictionary definitions, e.g. 'reassurance is to restore confidence, to remove the fears or doubts of' (verb)
Operational	Researchable definition 'reassurance is a purposeful attempt to restore confidence'
Empirical indicator	An instrument used to measure the concept, e.g. how would we know a patient is reassured?

another discipline or field of study and transposing it to a new field of study. During this process, the concept should be redefined to 'fit' the new area in which it is to be applied (Walker & Avant 1995). Concept synthesis is the process of developing concepts from observation in clinical practice or from other forms of evidence. Walker and Avant (1995) describe this process as starting from scratch. When concepts do exist, like reassurance, but may be abstract or lack clarity, a concept analysis may be undertaken. Concept analysis involves examination of the characteristics or attributes of the concept in question (see Ch. 5 for discussion of concept analysis).

The other form of propositional statement is referred to as a relational proposition or statement. As implied by the name, these statements are always concerned with two or more concepts. They are more complex in that they range from those that simply describe the existence of a relationship between two concepts to those that describe the direction of the relationship, or predict the relationship and conditions under which the relationship may or may not occur (see Table 4.4 for types and examples) (Fawcett & Downs 1992, McKenna 1997, Meleis 1997, Walker & Avant 1995). Relational propositions or statements, therefore, can generate descriptive, explanatory or predictive theory. For example, an existence relational statement generates descriptive theory, as it is merely concerned with the existence of a relationship between two concepts. A directional relational statement generates explanatory theory, as it explains the relationship, and a causal or deterministic relational statement generates predictive theory, as it makes a prediction about the relationship between the concepts.

As can be seen from Table 4.4, many relational propositions are predictive and, generally, the more developed they are, the more likely they are to be able to lead to predictive theory. It is also worth noting that a proposition may be more than one type at a time. As Walker and Avant (1995) note, most relational statements are probabilistic as well as being concurrent or contingent, and so on. Following the process of theory generation, hypotheses and research questions can be derived and tested by further research studies.

THEORY-VALIDATING RESEARCH

According to Chinn and Kramer (1999), once a theory has been constructed, by whatever means and to whatever level, it is possible to undertake a process of validating it by undertaking research. The overall purpose is to determine whether the theory depicts reality. This is usually thought of as the deductive approach (general to the specific—see Ch. 1) and correlates with McKenna's (1997) theory testing research and Meleis' (1997) theory research theory strategy.

As Chinn and Kramer (1999) and McKenna (1997) claim, the whole of a theory cannot be tested at one time. Therefore, concepts and propositions

Table 4.4 Relational propositions

Proposition type	Definition
Existence	Statement that a relationship exists, e.g. there is a relationship between anxiety and pain
Strength	Indicates how strong the relationship is between the concepts, e.g. there is a strong relationship between anxiety and pain
Shape	Reflects whether the shape of the relationship is linear or curvilinear, e.g. an increase in anxiety associated with an increase in pain is a linear relationship
Causal/deterministic	One concept is said to 'always' cause the other—there are few causal relationships in social and behavioural sciences
Probabilistic (e.g. stochastic)	The probability that one concept causes the other, e.g. anxiety is likely to lead to an increase in pain
Concurrent	If one concept occurs, then so does the other. There may be no statement of a causal relationship, just that the concepts occur together, e.g. poor health and poor living conditions occur together
Conditional/contingent	A relationship exists between two concepts but only in the presence of a third, e.g. hope enhances well-being but only in a supportive environment
Time ordered	When a relationship exists between two concepts but a time factor exists, e.g. intramuscular analgesia relieves pain after 20 minutes
Necessary	One and only one concept can lead to the other, e.g. only *Salmonella typhi* causes typhoid fever
Substitutional	The degree of certainty with which something will happen, e.g. *Streptococcus viridens* and *Staphylococcus epidermis* can both cause infective endocarditis
Sufficient	The first and second concepts are related regardless of anything else, e.g. hope will arise in a person following loss regardless of whether that person wills it
Direction	Specifies the direction of the relationship, either positively or negatively, or unknown. If both concepts increase or decrease in the same direction, then the relationship is positive. If one concept increases and the other decreases, then the relationship is negative, e.g. anxiety is positively related to pain
Symmetry	Asymmetrical is a one-way relationship and symmetrical is a two-way one, e.g. if an increase in anxiety is associated with increased pain but never the other way, it is asymmetrical

*The examples are hypothetical and no claim is made as to their truth value are extracted from the theory and tested in a particular research situation following identification of empiric indicators. Usually only one or two relational statements are tested in a single study. Basically, theory drives the research questions or hypotheses, and the findings from the subsequent study modify or inform the theory.

The theory to be tested may have been taken from another discipline. The researcher can choose to test the concepts in the original theory without changing or adapting them in any way for the nursing milieu. This is what is widely known as borrowing theory and, strictly speaking, corresponds with the theory research theory strategy. The findings of the study may indicate the original theory needs modification or adaptation.

An alternative approach that has been used in nursing concerns adapting and modifying theories from other disciplines for use in nursing situations. Although it does not exactly constitute theory testing, as it is usually used by theorists rather than researchers, it is worth considering given it could be considered as a precursor to the theory research theory strategy. Meleis (1997) identifies this as the theory practice theory strategy. During the process, it is discovered that the concepts of the original or parent theory need modifying or adaptation to better represent the practice situation. Having undertaken the adaptation or modification, there is potential for testing in nursing. This strategy, according to Meleis (1997) has been widely used in nursing. An example is Peplau's (1952) theory of interpersonal relations in nursing that was based on psychoanalytical theory. The original concepts of psychoanalytical theory were used as a framework for describing and explaining mental health nursing practice.

Some also 'regard these as 'borrowed' theories, but Stevens-Barnum (1998) disagrees and argues that adaptation and modification for nursing justifies these being described as 'shared' knowledge.

Activity 4.6

Try to list some areas of your practice that draw on theories from other disciplines. Do you think they have been adapted from the original theory or have they remained unchanged?

A further point concerns what McKenna (1997) describes as theory-framed research. In this situation, the researcher uses a theory to frame the study. Using a theoretical framework helps define the parameters of the study and guides all stages of the research process from literature review to data analysis and presentation of findings (Parahoo 1997). An example cited by Parahoo (1997) is the study of Jemmott and Jemmott (1991) who used the theory of reasoned action as a framework for their study on condom use among a group of black women in a USA inner city university. The theory considers the relationship between attitudes, beliefs, intentions, subjective norms and behaviours. In this example, the researchers used these theory components to review the literature, generate hypotheses and guide the structure of the questions used in data collection. Although the original intention may not have been to test the theory, the subsequent findings can lead to deductions about its effectiveness.

Activity 4.7

Consider an area of your practice that interests you or that has potential for investigation.
Try to identify a theory that you might use to frame a potential study.

It is important to note here that theories can vary in their potential to be tested. What this means is that some theories do not have well-developed concepts or propositions. This is an accusation that has been levelled at grand nursing theories that have a high number of assumptions, concepts that are abstract and have not been defined, and a limited number of propositions. Although some grand nursing theories are better developed than others, for example Orem (1995), others remain at a high level of abstraction and testing of these theories has been difficult. McKenna (1997) argues the best that can be done with grand nursing theories is to evaluate their potential impact on practice and education. For this reason, he has classed this as theory-evaluation research as opposed to theory testing.

Nevertheless, as indicated in Chapter 3, there has been greater activity recently in developing middle range theories from grand nursing theories. These are designed to test aspects of the grand theory as part of the process of validation or testing. Even though it may not be possible for all aspects of grand nursing theory to be tested, Chinn and Kramer (1999) claim incomplete testing does not mean the theory is not sound. If research studies concerning testable aspects of the theory have been conducted over time and in various situations, then some confidence in the theory is justified.

Activity 4.8

Consider the grand nursing theory or model that you may be using in clinical practice.
Can you think of any of its aspects that might be tested in a research study?

As hypotheses must include a relationship between at least two variables, research designs in theory-validating research are usually experimental, quasi-experimental or correlational. The subsequent findings should say something about the theory. However, theory-validating research can also be descriptive or exploratory in nature. In this instance, hypotheses may not be stated and research questions are developed that implicitly signify relationships between the variables as opposed to hypotheses that state the relationships explicitly. The usual designs for these studies are descriptive and correlational.

According to McKenna (1997, 197), findings from theory validating or testing research may lead to:

- support for the validity of the theory
- refutation of the validity of the theory
- adaptation or revision of the theory
- formulation of a new theory (note: theory testing may lead to theory generation).

Finally, in this section, some discussion of Meleis' (1997) 'integrated approach' is worthy of mention. This appears to have replaced her 'practice theory research theory' strategy discussed in the 1991 edition of her book. Essentially, this approach argues that not only do practice, theory and research have a role to play in the development of theory, but so do clinicians,

Table 4.5 From phenomenon to theory

Stages	Definition
Taking in	Attention grabbing—something in practice attracts your attention either through observation, sensing or mental activity or personal involvement Developing a hunch Attention giving—careful examination of situations or events that may illuminate the phenomenon under consideration
Describing the phenomenon	The process of defining the phenomenon under consideration
Labelling	To reduce the phenomenon that is usually described in a paragraph to a concept or statement: ● It should be precise ● It should have only one idea ● It should be consistent in its meaning.
Concept development (see Ch. 5)	Stages of concept development [see Ch. 5 for Walker and Avant (1995) and Rodgers' (2000) framework for concept analysis]
Statement development	Explanations related to the phenomenon are provided. The explanations link the concepts, antecedents, consequences and assumptions Statements are provided to describe, explain, prescribe or predict Propositional statements, either relational or nonrelational, are developed
Explicating assumptions	Reflection, analysis and questioning of implicit and explicit assumptions
Sharing and communicating	Sharing and communicating theorising with colleagues in the form of conferences, publications, seminars, journal clubs and so on

theorists and researchers. Meleis (1997) claims that nursing as a human and caring science cannot be fully explored using the other strategies she identified (see Table 4.2) as they are carried out in isolation from each other. Thus, she recommends an integrated approach that begins in clinical practice, leads to theory that is tested by research, and results in modified, refuted, validated or new theory. In advocating integration, Meleis (1997) contends multiple sources of data should be accessed, including skills and tools from clinical practice, research, reflective clinical diaries and descriptive journals. A variety of research designs are also a significant component of this strategy. She considers previous experiences are part of the nursing perspective and should be considered when generating and validating theory.

Meleis (1997) proposes there are stages and processes that are useful when involved with theorising, whether it simply involves theory framing or the development of theory. However, she acknowledges there is no one way of developing theories. The process is not linear, stages can happen simultaneously and there is no guarantee that, after years of work, the subsequent theory will reflect reality in any way. The stages and processes as represented by Meleis (1997) are summarised in Table 4.5 as an example of one way of developing theory from a phenomenon. This process is demonstrated by the following hypothetical example.

Activity 4.9

While reading the hypothetical example below, try to identify the stages described by Meleis (1997).

EXEMPLAR

At some time in history, somebody noticed that sick or ill people who were confined to bed developed wounds or sores. This phenomenon did not just happen in hospitals, but also occurred in people's homes and they have even been noted in unearthed Egyptian mummies. It was noticed that all sick people did not develop these sores. Initially, these sores were termed 'bed sores' or 'decubitus ulcers' because a key characteristic appeared to be confinement to bed. Decubitus derives from the Latin *decumbere* meaning to 'lie down'. However, it was noted that this phenomenon did not just occur in those who were lying down. People who were confined in a sitting position also developed these sores. They developed in particular places on the body such as the sacrum, shoulders, elbows and heels. They varied in their severity but, the longer somebody was confined, the worse they seemed to get. However, as the concept was investigated further, significant characteristics were identified. These sores appeared to occur mainly over bony prominences of the body and they tended to occur in people who were immobile. They were more prevalent in the older population or those who were debilitated. This led to the hypothesis that it was not confinement to bed that caused these sores but unrelieved pressure on the bony prominences of the body. Thus, the phenomenon was relabelled 'pressure sore' as the common denominator in the development of these sores was pressure. The emerging theory was that there was a causal relationship between unrelieved pressure and pressure sores.

The nature of pressure sores was delineated further by the development of classification systems that enabled description and established consistency in describing the concept.

The other concept in the relationship, 'pressure', was addressed. What kind of pressure had to be exerted for a pressure sore to occur? How long did the pressure have to be unrelieved before a pressure sore developed? Were there any factors that mitigated the amount of pressure needed for a pressure sore to occur? These questions were addressed by referring to the science of physics and through research. The nature of the pressure was that exerted by the weight of the person on the skin, soft tissue and bone. If the pressure exerted was greater than the normal capillary filling pressure, estimated at 32mmHg, then localised ischaemia occurred, leading eventually to necrosis and ulceration. It was also found that certain factors, such as age and artificial lowering of blood pressure, resulted in reduced capillary filling pressure. It was concluded that there is a variation in people's capillary filling pressure; therefore, the time needed for ischaemia to develop would also vary. Several other factors, such as general health, nutritional status, poor blood supply and body weight, appeared to be contingent, although pressure is the final common pathway.

Having delineated the concepts and established a causal relationship between them, intervention strategies aimed at controlling the phenomena were proposed. Based on the length of time pressure could be exerted before tissue damage began to occur, prevention strategies focused on altering the person's position and relieving pressure. This was initially calculated at 2-hour intervals but was largely based on normal capillary filling pressure. Some people continued to develop pressure sores. Thus, standard interventions were not always adequate and there was a need to identify those people who were most at risk. Risk assessment tools were identified and have become an important factor in identifying prevention strategies.

Much work continues on prevention and management of pressure sores, now relabelled pressure ulcers, given the chronic nature of the wound and its relationship with ulceration.

You may have noticed that the stages outlined by Meleis (1997) did not occur in a linear fashion in this example. Phenomena that have been identified, described and labelled are often revisited, refined and relabelled as development occurs. What is clear, then, is that theory development is complex and the knowledge developed is always subject to change.

SUMMARY

This chapter was concerned with the relationship between theory, research and practice. It was proposed that not only do these concepts form three core elements in nursing, but that they are mutually interrelated and interdependent. Research was proposed as being the link between theory and practice. It was suggested that a lack of true understanding of the interrelationship between the three concepts exists and to some extent can be located in the hierarchical relationship between theory and practice, and between research and practice. The traditional view of the theory–practice relationship is one where greater importance was attached to theory whose purpose was to guide and direct nursing practice. Similarly, research is seen at times to be an elitist activity far removed from and not always relevant to practice.

A brief overview of the position of research in nursing was offered with an emphasis on the need for approaches other than experimental designs. It was also proposed that with a broad conception of theory, there is potential for all research to be theory linked. Such an approach is advocated, as isolated research studies may not contribute to the development of the overall body of knowledge in nursing. Given the considerable effort needed to undertake a research project or study, it is suggested that such effort is wasted if it contributes little.

Chinn and Kramer's (1999) framework of theory generating and theory testing was utilised to structure the discussion on the possible relationships between theory, research and practice. Those of McKenna (1997) and Meleis (1997) were integrated to demonstrate the similarities and differences in how the relationships can be conceived.

Finally, Meleis' (1997) proposal for an integrated strategy was outlined and her strategy for theory development presented. Her arguments for such a strategy are bound in the practice-based nature of nursing, and the belief that no one strategy will address the questions or phenomena of interest to nursing.

5

How do we use concepts in practice?

INTRODUCTION

In Chapters 3 and 4, concepts as elements of theory were explored. It was emphasised that, without concepts and conceptual clarity, meaningful and useful theory generation and theory testing is not possible. In this chapter, the nature of concepts is revisited and some discussion of the importance of conceptual clarity is presented. The value of concept analysis is outlined and two frameworks for analysis are presented. The place of concept analysis in the interrelationships between theory, research and practice is delineated. The value of using published concept analyses to enhance individual practice is examined and activities related to the concept of hope are included as an exemplar. The chapter concludes with some self-directed activities for the reader.

INTENDED LEARNING OUTCOMES

At the end of this chapter you will be able to:

1. offer a definition of the term concept
2. discuss the value of conceptual clarity for nursing
3. describe how to undertake a concept analysis
4. critically appraise literature relating to the concept of hope and analyse its relevance to a practice scenario.

WHAT ARE CONCEPTS?

According to Chinn and Kramer (1999, 54), a concept is 'a complex mental formulation of our experience'. Our experiences shape our perceptions of the world in that we learn through them and, through this learning, we attach meaning. Language is the medium through which we communicate our experiences, our perception of them and the meaning we attach to them. Language is how we try to achieve understanding of others and they of us.

Yet, language is, in itself, complex and contextual. In different societies, cultures and even subgroups within these, different meanings can be attached to the words used. For example, if communicating with a patient, you may use words or terms that would have a common meaning within the wider society to describe a condition or intervention, whereas you may use more scientific or professional terms to discuss the same issue with colleagues. Similarly, a word may have several different meanings, depending on the context in which it is used. For instance, 'glasses' is a term used to describe drinking utensils, but is also commonly used when referring to spectacles. It is in the context of its usage and implied purpose that meaning is conveyed.

The process by which we learn to understand the words and the context in which they are being used begins as a child and can be referred to as conceptualisation. For example, a child will be able to identify and name a dog. However, when they first learn to communicate through language, they may label all animals they see as dogs. This is because they have not yet learned to discriminate between the particular attributes of different animals. As they develop and learn through their experience, not only can they identify the features that are common to animals, but they can also use the differences as a means of discrimination. This is the beginning of conceptualisation, when an individual can label the things they see and also ascribe meaning to them.

Conceptual meaning, claim Chinn and Kramer (1999), is created by considering the word used to describe the concept, an encounter with the object/thing itself and the feelings associated with it. If we take our previous example of dog, the use of the word 'dog' conjures an image of a specific animal. This image may vary depending on our previous encounters with dogs, e.g. a poodle or a German shepherd. For some, associated feelings may be fear and anxiety, while for others, feelings of warmth and companionship may be generated.

This demonstrates that, even what could be conceived as a concrete concept, such as 'dog', carries with it differing perceptions. As all concepts are located on a continuum from concrete to abstract, imagine the difficulties when faced with more abstract concepts such as love or hate. The possibilities for varied perceptions and attributed meanings are much greater, thus making description, recognition and understanding of the concepts more complex.

Activity 5.1
Note down some concepts commonly used in nursing. How do you know you are using the concept in the same way as others? Are there any examples of concepts that have proved to be ambiguous or difficult to grasp?

THE NEED FOR CONCEPTUAL CLARITY

As with everyday life, concepts in nursing range on a continuum from concrete to abstract. Concrete concepts, such as a person's height, weight, blood pressure and temperature, can be directly measured and are useful in diagnosis and prognostics. Abstract concepts, such as pain, suffering and compassion, are not directly measurable and are, therefore, relative and can only be inferred. The problem this poses in nursing is that the patient's perception of these may be at variance with that of the nurse.

For example, we often see 'maintain patient's privacy and dignity' on a care plan, but there is little indication of what the nurse needs to do in order to achieve this. Maintaining patients' privacy and dignity is open to interpretation by individual nurses, based on their unique experience of the concepts and their understanding of them. In practice, this can lead to inconsistency in the quality and standard of care being delivered. The existence and potential for inconsistency could be said to be evident in the perceived need to identify benchmarks for this area of fundamental and essential care (Department of Health 2001a).

Conceptual clarity is, therefore, of paramount importance if, as a discipline, nursing aspires to provide consistent and meaningful care to our patients. Part of the process of clarifying the concepts we use in practice is through concept analysis. This can be evidenced by the plethora of literature related to concepts, such as hope, reassurance, trust, caring, suffering, and fatigue, to name but a few.

However, conceptual clarity is also significant in the development, refinement, evaluation and use of theory. As discussed in Chapter 3, concepts are often described as the building blocks of theory. All theories are made up of concepts but the level of abstraction of the concepts varies. In evaluating a theory for possible use in practice, be it a nursing theory or one borrowed from another discipline, part of the process is to examine the concepts for clarity. This enables the practitioner to determine not only whether the concepts are at a level of concreteness whereby the concept can be measured but also to gain some idea of whether the theorist's conceptual meaning is congruent with the practitioner's area of practice.

In terms of theory development, the first level, according to Dickoff et al (1968), is factor-isolating or naming (see Ch. 3). Naming or isolating the concepts to be used in the theory is essential to its ultimate clarity and

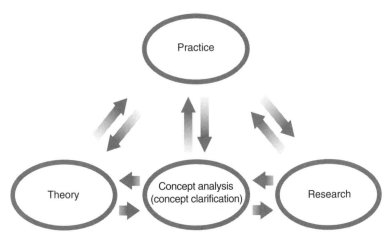

Figure 5.1   The interrelationship between theory, practice, research and conceptual clarification.

utility in practice. For example, if a practitioner wants to investigate 'anxiety' in patients, the first step would be to clarify what is meant by the concept in the context in which it is being used. Similarly, in refining a theory, the investigator may wish to re-examine the conceptual meaning of a concept in order to ensure its adequacy in describing the experience under investigation. Thus, it is argued that conceptual clarity is essential to practice, theory and research in nursing. Figure 5.1 represents the relationship between conceptual clarity, theory, research and practice.

WHAT IS THE VALUE OF CONCEPT ANALYSIS?

In the previous section, the usefulness of conceptual clarity was emphasised. The question remains as to how we achieve conceptual clarity. One approach is to undertake a concept analysis. There are several reasons for such an undertaking:

- distinguishing between a concept's defining attributes and its irrelevant attributes
- identifying pertinent areas for research
- improving nursing practice
- refining ambiguous concepts in a theory
- clarifying overused, vague or abstract concepts
- developing a rigorous process for operationalising variables

(Kramer 1993, Walker & Avant 1995).

Additionally, undertaking a concept analysis helps to develop skills of critical inquiry and critical thinking in that it involves purposeful and rigorous investigation of a concept. In order to investigate the true meaning of a concept and its application and relevance to nursing practice, theory or research, the nurse requires the skills to appraise the evidence critically, analyse the available data and synthesise the results into a meaningful whole.

Any attempt to analyse a concept of interest is not to be taken lightly as it can be time-consuming and frustrating. Paley (1996) suggests that such an undertaking is vacuous, as concept analysis can become a mere exercise in semantics if authors do not clearly identify the reasons for their decisions in the process of concept analysis. However, as the discipline of nursing matures and its knowledge base becomes more established, the quality of published concept analyses has shown a marked improvement in both presentation and explication of the processes undertaken. In addition, more refined and advanced techniques for attaining conceptual clarity and adequacy have been discussed and utilised to enhance the utility of concept analysis (Morse 1995, Morse et al 1996). For example, following analysis of a concept, its critical attributes can be tested in practice by undertaking research. Such a process will enable the validation of the concept for use with different groups and in different contexts. This process can lead to refinement or adaptation of the concept, or it may lead to the development of middle range theory (see Ch. 3 on middle range theory).

Activity 5.2

Make a list of concepts that have been problematic in your practice. Try to identify aspects of their use that have been difficult.

At this point, it would be useful to discuss briefly how a concept analysis might be undertaken. There are several methods for doing this (Rodgers 2000, Walker & Avant 1995, Wilson 1963). It is worth noting that, whatever method is chosen, the outcomes of any analysis can only be tentative, as concepts can change with use and as situations and practice develop. Additionally, two people may draw different conclusions when investigating the same concept, owing to the realm of data analysed, their skills of critical thinking and the manner in which they synthesise the material. For the purposes of this chapter, the models proposed by Walker and Avant (1995) and Rodgers (2000) will be described.

WALKER AND AVANT'S METHOD

Walker & Avant (1995, 39) propose eight steps in concept analysis:

1. Select a concept of interest.
2. Determine the aim(s).

3. Identify all the uses of the concept.
4. Determine the defining critical attributes.
5. Construct a model case.
6. Construct additional cases.
7. Identify antecedents and consequences.
8. Define empirical referents.

They state that these steps are not always sequential and may be simultaneous, and former steps may be revised as new data come to light. They emphasise the importance of choosing a concept carefully and examining the aims of the analysis. The overarching aim should be to contribute to the development of nursing knowledge. However, the nurse will need to be clear about what they will do with the analysis once it is complete, as this may influence decisions during the process. As the work will take a significant amount of effort and time, it should be something of interest or something that has puzzled or intrigued the nurse.

When identifying the uses of the concept, these should be both implicit and explicit, and should also cover the realm of physical, psychological and social uses. It is also useful to search for different uses of the concept in more than one discipline. For example, do physiotherapists use the same concept in a different manner to nursing or is there a common understanding across disciplines? In order to search for the whole variety of uses of a concept, sources of data can be literature of the discipline in question as well as that of others; popular literature, such as magazines; music; film, and multimedia sources, such as letters, historical artefacts and the Internet. It is important at this stage not to discard any uses, as this may limit the analysis. It may be that, later in the process, clarification will be needed as to why certain uses are being discarded. Walker and Avant (1995) state that, at this stage, some uses that are not quite 'the real thing' may be discovered. It is important to note these, as they may facilitate the construction of borderline cases later in the analysis. This is probably the lengthiest and most time-consuming step, but being thorough at this stage will determine the overall rigour of the analysis. The fourth step of this method is to define the attributes of the concept, that is, what characteristics demonstrate the concept? Identification of these criteria may not produce a long list, but should include those attributes that demonstrate the presence of the concept under investigation.

Steps five and six are related to constructing cases that will demonstrate clearly what is or is not the concept, including examples of cases that are related but are not actually the concept. Cases can be constructed or may be case studies from observations or the literature. Walker and Avant (1995) identify the need to discuss borderline, related, contrary, invented and illegitimate cases in order to clearly delineate the parameters of the concept being analysed.

In the penultimate stage, antecedents and consequences of the concept are identified. Antecedents are those events or incidents that must be present for the concept to happen. Consequences are the outcome of the concept having occurred. It is important to note that antecedents and consequences cannot also be critical attributes.

The final stage, naming empirical referents, is the operationalisation of the concept, that is, how the concept can be observed or measured.

The method utilised by Walker and Avant is quantitative in nature, and has been criticised for being reductionist and not taking account of change over time. However, they refute this, as they do not support the idea of concept analysis being an end point, but consider it a part of critical inquiry that is larger than the analysis itself.

Activity 5.3

Reflect upon the concepts you identified in Activity 5.2.
Do you think undertaking a concept analysis would help to clarify the difficulties noted?

RODGERS' METHOD

Rodgers (2000) has modified the process originally proposed by Walker and Avant (1983), and proposes a method of concept analysis that has an inductive and evolutionary process that helps to clarify the current status of a concept. She states that the current meaning of a concept is influenced by its history and that investigating this evolutionary cycle helps to develop the knowledge base of nursing.

Rodgers believes that concepts become associated with particular attributes through socialisation, that is, public discourse and common usage of the concepts in practice. Thus, any clarification that uncovers such an evolution in terms of a concept's significance, use and application can only enhance its use in future encounters. A concept may be enhanced by an understanding of its explanatory powers and its relevance to a variety of practice settings. Rodgers' method of concept analysis is more related to uncovering common usage, rather than applying strict criteria to it.

Rodgers (2000, 85) describes six activities in the evolutionary method that may not proceed in a linear fashion. These stages are:

- identify the concept of interest and surrogate terms
- identify and decide upon an appropriate realm of data
- collect data to identify attributes and the contextual basis of the concept
- analyse the data
- identify an exemplar
- identify implications.

Similar to Walker and Avant's (1995) method, the first stage is identifying and naming the concept of interest. However, Rodgers emphasises the importance of identifying surrogate terms as several terms may serve as expressions of a concept. This can be a problem related to linguistics rather than with the concept itself, and identifying surrogate terms replaces the need to construct borderline, contrary, invented and illegitimate cases. This activity can reveal different perspectives on a concept across disciplines or over time.

The second phase highlights the importance of choosing an appropriate realm or sample of data from which the analysis develops. She reiterates Walker and Avant's argument for a systematic trawl of a wide range of data, but additionally emphasises the need to address a broad time frame to facilitate the examination of changes over time. It is this emphasis that highlights the contextual and historical relevance of the analysis. The realm chosen will be influenced by the purpose of undertaking the analysis and the desired outcomes.

The third phase is related to collecting and managing the data. Rodgers stresses that an inductive approach to concept analysis is required, thus attributes of the concept should be identified from the literature, rather than model cases constructed as illustrations. She also contends that the contextual basis of the concept needs to be identified from the data. For example, what socio-political or temporal variations occur in the descriptions of the concept under investigation? The focus is an understanding of the situations in which the concept is used and how perspectives across contexts may vary. Additional surrogate terms may be identified at this stage.

The fourth stage of analysis entails allowing the characteristics of the concept to emerge from the data. Rodgers notes that the greatest challenge in the analysis is avoiding preconceived notions of what the analyst thinks the concept should be. Consequently, she suggests that the analysis be left until the end of data collection rather than the usual qualitative concurrent analysis providing direction for future data collection. Thematic analysis is carried out until a cohesive and relevant system of descriptors is generated.

The fifth stage involves identifying rather than constructing an exemplar. Rodgers states that inability to do so reveals important information about the development of the concept.

The final stage of Rodgers' framework is identifying the implications of the concept analysis. Rather than providing a definitive answer to questions about the concepts, this stage gives direction to additional inquiry and to enhance the continuing cycle of concept development.

Concept analysis is a time-consuming activity and you may not have the time or the resources to undertake one. To help you to answer questions related to ill-defined concepts you may encounter in practice, an alternative strategy might be to review published concept analyses and research. In the following section, Walker and Avant's (1995) framework will be used to direct activities using published material to consider the concept of hope.

HOPE

Activity 5.4

Read the following literature (see References at end for full details) and carry out the activities in relation to the scenario below:
Benzein & Saveman (1998), Cutliffe & Herth (2002a, 2002b, 2002c), Haase et al (1992), Herth (1990), Kylmä & Vehviläinen-Julkunen (1997), Morse & Doberneck (1995), Penrod & Morse (1997), Rustøen & Hanestad (1998) and Stephenson (1991).
Mr Anderson is a 59-year-old man with peripheral vascular disease who has been admitted to your ward for investigations into severe intermittent claudication in his right leg. He had a femoro-popliteal bypass graft 1 year ago, but his symptoms have recurred in the last 3 months. He has been unable to work for the last 2 months, as his job as a hospital porter requires a lot of walking. He tells the staff nurse that he had given up smoking over 2 years ago and he had thought that this would have stopped the progress of his disease. He confides that he is terrified that he will lose his leg and how that will impact on his future.

Activity 5.5

In the above scenario, identify the antecedents of the concept of hope.

Benzein and Saveman (1998) consider the antecedents of hope to be the presence of stressful stimuli, loss, a life-threatening situation and a temptation to despair. Similarly, Stephenson (1991) identifies loss, a life-threatening situation and despair, but argues that a difficult decision or challenge could also be possible antecedents to hope.

In the scenario, Mr Anderson has certainly been exposed to stressful stimuli and anticipated loss not only in terms of the potential loss of a limb, but associated losses in terms of personal autonomy, loss of control and employment. It is difficult to assess at this stage whether he perceives this to be a life-threatening situation, but he perceives the disease process has not been arrested. The fact that he has confided he is terrified indicates a temptation to despair.

Activity 5.6

What action should the nurse take to foster hope in Mr Anderson?

Rustøen and Hanestad (1998) claim that helping an ill person to maintain hope and avoid hopelessness is a major task for the professional nurse. According to Benzein and Saveman (1998) and Stephenson (1991), the critical attributes of hope include future-orientation, positive expectation, intentionality, activity, realism, goal-setting and interconnectedness.

Haase et al (1992) add that a feeling of uncertainty may exist, while Herth (1990) suggests that a spiritual base and personal attributes may be pertinent.

The nurse should have knowledge of these critical attributes so that nursing activities can be directed towards fostering rather than minimising hope in Mr Anderson (see Table 5.1). The literature appears to agree universally that interconnectedness encompasses meaningful relationships with others (Benzein & Saveman 1998, Herth 1990, Kylmä & Vehviläinen-Julkunen 1997, Penrod & Morse 1997, Rustøen & Hanestad 1998). In Mr Anderson's case, the nurse should, as part of assessment and care planning, evaluate his family and social support network and determine any spiritual needs he may have (Cutliffe & Herth 2002c). His family should be encouraged to participate actively in helping support Mr Anderson. Nursing staff should also be aware of the need to 'make time' for the patient and listen to fears and hopes. Even if the nurse finds it difficult to discuss Mr Anderson's fears with him, failure to do so can lead to feelings of isolation and poor self-worth.

Even if prognosis is poor, the nurse can help the patient to appreciate that they do have a future. One strategy for achieving this is to facilitate the patient setting attainable goals. An example in Mr Anderson's case might be to help him formulate the questions he might wish to put to the medical team about possible treatment options. Emotional support could help Mr Anderson to focus on his immediate future, as the long-term future is currently uncertain. It would be wrong for the nurse to determine goals on behalf of the patient as it would rush him in his endeavours.

Although having hope is seen as a positive coping strategy (Morse & Doberneck 1995) especially in times of uncertainty, the patient needs to have some positive expectations. However, these expectations must be realistic and not give the patient false hope. Nurses should be truthful in their interactions and should acknowledge that amputation might be a possible outcome. For example, it would not be helpful for the nurse to say 'I'm sure it won't come to that—don't worry'. The skilled nurse will also be able to help Mr Anderson to see some positive outcome even in a worse case scenario. For Mr Anderson this may mean exploring the possibility of full mobility and a return to employment following amputation.

Activity as a critical attribute is not limited to the physical aspects, and includes psychological activity that minimises introspection and withdrawal. For Mr Anderson it is likely that he will have bed-rest prescribed, but the nurse can ensure he remains as active as possible by encouraging both physical and psychological self-care.

Activity 5.7
What are the expected outcomes (consequences) of fostering hope in Mr Anderson?

Table 5.1 Nursing strategies that foster and hinder hope

Critical attributes	Hope-fostering strategies	Strategies that hinder hope
Interconnectedness	• Discuss individual value as a family member whether working or not • Use therapeutic touch • Monitor support network and reinforce availability of resources during and as treatment continues • Ascertain spiritual needs and access appropriate resource • 'Be there' for the patient and be prepared to listen to their story • Use light-heartedness when appropriate	• Patient isolation either physical/psychological/social/emotional/spiritual/cultural • Avoiding patients
Future orientation; attainable goals and intentionality	• Help the patient to identify immediate needs and set short-term goals to meet these; e.g. help the patient to identify and record his information needs, which can be used to consult with medical staff • Help the patient to ensure goals are focused and attainable • Provide emotional support and allow time for contemplation and re-examination	• Lack of skill in goal-setting • Lack of skills of communication • 'Doing for' the patient by setting goals and rushing the patient to make decisions • Not allowing time or interrupting contemplation
Uncertainty, realism and positive expectation	• Acknowledge perceived threat to patient • Discuss options in truthful manner, including possible negative outcomes • Give honest appraisal of progress towards goals • Revisit education needs • Discuss available resources	• Failure to acknowledge threat to patient • Telling lies to protect 'self' or patient • Failure to educate patient • Failure to evaluate progress
Activity	• See goal-setting above • Mental activity–can include distractors, e.g. reading/radio • Physical activity—promoting self-care to the maximum potential of the patient in the given context • Explore with the patient personal resources and coping strategies which have been used and have worked in the past	• Allowing patient to become bored or introspective • Inappropriately 'doing for' the patient and hindering ability to self-care

Although there is some disparity in the literature as to the outcomes or consequences of hope, there is some agreement that fostering hope leads to an increased ability to cope with difficult situations, develop new coping strategies and a sense of peace and renewal (Benzein & Saveman 1998). Others that have been postulated include an improved quality of life and physical well-being. However, this cannot be argued to be a universal consequence. In Mr Anderson's case, it is envisaged that the strategies discussed above would help him develop positive coping strategies and a level of acceptance of his situation that would enable him to face his future with renewed determination and stamina.

The above example demonstrates that accessing concept analyses and research related to hope can significantly enhance a nurse's understanding of the concept. This increased knowledge should equip the nurse with the skills to identify the patient that feels hopeless, and to determine appropriate actions or interventions to promote hope.

TRUST

Activity 5.8

Read the recommended literature (see References for full details) and scenario related to the concept of trust and, using the same process as that employed for hope, answer the questions below.

Hams (1997), Hupcey et al (2001), Johns (1996) and Meize-Grochowski (1984).

Mrs Jones who is 44 years old was admitted to your ward yesterday with an acute upper respiratory tract infection. She has had multiple sclerosis for 15 years and is wheelchair bound. Although she has had many hospital admissions over the years, this is the first time she has been admitted to your ward, as there were no beds available in her usual ward. At handover this morning, you were informed by the night staff that she was incontinent of urine during the night.

Having greeted Mrs Jones, you inform her that you will be caring for her during the day and you would like to discuss how this can be best planned. At first she does not respond and she appears to be upset. When you ask if something is wrong she says 'All I want is that someone responds when I ask to go to the toilet'.

Questions

1. Identify from the scenario what you consider to be the key elements of the concept of trust.
2. In this scenario, what are the factors for the nurse and the patient that will impact on the formation of a trusting relationship?
3. What activities could the nurse undertake to promote the patient's trust?
4. Outline how knowledge of activities to promote trust may influence your future practice.

SUMMARY

This chapter has demonstrated the need for conceptual clarity in nursing practice. Concept analysis as one way of achieving this was presented to develop the reader's understanding of its inherent value for theory generation and testing and, ultimately, its importance for practice and the development of practice theory. Rodgers' (2000) and Walker and Avant's (1995) methods for analysis were outlined as examples of frameworks utilised in nursing. For those who are unable to carry out their own concept analyses, the manner in which published analyses can be used to inform practice was presented using the concept of hope as an example.

The nature of nursing practice

In Section 2 professional issues that are of concern to nurses are explored. These include the nature of professional nursing practice and the concepts of profession, responsibility, accountability, autonomy and authority. Decision-making in nursing is presented and followed by an examination of how care is organised. The section concludes with an exploration of the notion of reflection.

SECTION CONTENTS

6

What is professional nursing practice?

INTRODUCTION

In Section 1, we reviewed the nature of philosophy, knowledge, theory and research, and explored how they have influenced and have been influenced by nursing. A recurring theme in Section 1 was the dominance of the positivist tradition, and its influence on both nursing practice and its evidence base. Another theme was that of nurses not valuing theory and research, and perceiving them to be irrelevant to their own everyday practice. However, any knowledge or theory must be seen in context and, in Section 2, we will endeavour to delineate how knowledge, theory and research informs practice and contemporary professional issues. In this chapter, the issue of professional nursing practice is discussed within the context of the changing health-care arena. The long-standing debate relating to whether nursing is really a profession is examined and related to the contemporary role of the nurse. The issues of responsibility, authority, autonomy, accountability and expanding roles are discussed in relation to the Code of Professional Conduct.

INTENDED LEARNING OUTCOMES

By the end of this chapter you will:

1. be able to debate whether nursing is a profession
2. articulate the differences between responsibility, authority, autonomy and accountability

3. be able to discuss critically the implications of expanding nursing practice
4. be able to reflect upon the implications of the Code of Professional Conduct for your own practice.

Activity 6.1

Do you consider yourself to be a member of a profession?
What criteria are you using when trying to decide upon this issue?
How did you select these criteria?

IS NURSING A PROFESSION?

The Nursing and Midwifery Council (NMC) is the regulatory body for nursing midwifery and health visiting. Its remit is to protect the public through professional standards (NMC 2002) and implicit in this statement is the assumption that nursing is a profession. However, this premise needs to be explored if the nature of professional nursing practice is to be discussed in any meaningful way.

Sociologists have long debated what it means to be a profession. The functionalist approach identifies characteristics evident in an ideal type of profession and then measures an occupational group against these criteria. There is some disagreement amongst sociologists as to which criteria should be used, but several criteria are commonly noted. For our purposes, the criteria for a profession cited by Taylor et al (1995) will be used as they include those generally agreed upon as being the archetypal characteristics of a profession:

- a systematic knowledge base with prolonged training
- a service ideal—a strong commitment to clients' well-being
- a high degree of autonomy and control through self-regulation and standard setting.

If we examine these principles, it could be said, at first glance, that nursing meets all the requirements. The education of nurses is established within higher education and has a firm knowledge base, which is currently being expanded with the rapid increase in nursing research. A strong service ideal is apparent, with the client's well-being and best interests being at the very core of nursing practice. The Code of Professional Conduct (NMC 2002) clearly delineates its values, and states that nurses must protect and support not only individual clients and patients, but also the health of the wider community. Finally, the NMC has clear regulatory powers over the registration and ongoing education of nurses, and sets clear guidelines and standards for practice.

However, some might argue that, when investigating the principles more closely, nursing falls short of these ideals. Walsh (2000) states that, although nursing has a specialised body of knowledge, it has drawn heavily on the social and biomedical sciences for its theoretical underpinning and thus does not have its own unique knowledge base. Leddy and Pepper (1998), however, contend that, while nursing initially derived its knowledge base by the application of theories from other disciplines, in recent years, nursing theorists have developed frameworks and models that are uniquely relevant to nursing. Moreover, theory-building research is helping to form a systematic knowledge base. Yet, their argument assumes that theory building and theory testing using the scientific method is the valid path to knowledge, and this in itself has been challenged, as was discussed previously in Chapter 1.

It could also be argued that it is not enough for a profession to have a recognised body of knowledge and a specialised education to transmit that knowledge, if nurses do not apply it in practice. The United Kingdom Central Council for Nursing, Midwifery and Health Visiting (UKCC) acknowledged that nurse education has, in the past, ill-equipped the nurse for the levels of clinical decision-making required of them in contemporary clinical practice and recommended that this be addressed in new programmes of study (UKCC 1999). This suggests that, while nursing may be developing the required body of knowledge, many individual nurses are a long way off using relevant clinical reasoning and decision-making skills in practice. Additionally, Walsh (2000) states that, although nurse education is now in higher education, the majority of nurses register at diploma, rather than graduate level and that many nurses are hostile to the notion of nursing becoming an all-graduate profession. If this is the case, it would seem that not all nurses aspire to professional status.

It is hard to argue against the second criterion of having a strong service ideal. Nursing has always had the welfare of its patients as the core of its purpose but, because of this, it is seen by many, both within and outside of nursing, as a vocation rather than a professional career. The notion of nursing as a vocation, along with historically being a female occupation, has led to poor financial rewards. The satisfaction of knowing that patients have benefited from nursing care has been seen to be reward enough. However, the rising expectations of women in the workforce, an increase in men in nursing and the increasingly complex nature of nursing has led to a dissatisfaction with the status quo and the demand for higher financial reward for nurses. The current shortage of nurses and the retention difficulties presently faced in both the NHS and independent sectors of health care might not reflect as strong a service ideal as might be expected of a profession. However, this may be an unfair criticism of nursing, as well-established professions such as medicine and the law have a strong commitment to the client, yet also reap the benefits of a high financial reward.

This aspect is also related to the third criterion of a high degree of autonomy and control, which will now be discussed in the light of the historical development of nursing. Nursing first gained registration status with the Nursing Registration Acts of 1919 and the setting up of the General Nursing Council (GNC). Even so, the GNC had little power, and any decisions it made required the approval of the Minister of Health and the Houses of Parliament. Nurses were still seen as handmaidens to the medical profession and had little power to influence care provision. The UKCC and National Boards later took over the regulation of nursing, and have now been replaced by the Nursing and Midwifery Council that took up its powers in April 2002. The NMC, and previously the UKCC and National Boards, manages the regulation of nursing by guaranteeing competence and ethical practice through education and standards, but also has the power to remove unfit nurses from the register. Thus, from a broad perspective, nursing does meet the requirement of a profession to have a high degree of autonomy and control. We will discuss later in this chapter whether the same level of control is afforded to individual nurses in their everyday practice.

At this stage, perhaps it is worth noting that the elements of what constitutes a profession have usually been abstracted from established, male dominated professions, such as medicine and the law (McNeil & Townley 1986), and this functionalist approach to the professions has its critics. For example, Illich (1977) contended that society was not served well by professions and that they are in fact self-serving groups who use the guise of professionalism to gain status and financial reward. The Weberian approach also contends that professions are primarily occupational groups who have controlled the market in such a way that they can maximise their rewards, and that self-government prevents external scrutiny of their affairs (Haralambos & Holborn 2000). The historical evolution of the medical profession prior to state control has resulted in it having a high degree of power and dominance within the health-care arena and nursing has always been subordinate to it. Thus, it could be argued from this perspective that nursing's aspirations towards being a profession and its desire to be more 'scientific' are simply mimicry and another illustration of its subservience to the medical profession.

Macdonald (1997) discusses the 'professional project', whereby groups continually struggle to enhance their status as a profession. Macdonald argues that, to achieve professional status, a group needs to accomplish social closure; define their jurisdiction and their area of expertise, and then they have to monopolise that professional expertise. The final stage is to attain respectability. In this model, nursing has only just started in its attempts to be recognised as a profession. While nursing can stipulate entry criteria to the profession as a means of social closure, it is battling against government attempts to widen the entry gates in a bid to increase the number of nurses. It is still struggling to describe what nursing is and how it differs from other disciplines. This failure to gain consensus on what is unique to nursing is another stumbling block to attaining professional status and, although nursing is valued by society, it clearly does not have the same standing as medicine.

Porter (1992) notes that an increase in managerialism has been deemed by some nurses as a way of gaining professional standing. However, he also maintains that, while nurses in managerial positions may have gained power, prestige and in many cases financial reward, this should not be mistaken for gaining professional status. He contends that, when nurses' autonomy is dictated by a nursing hierarchy, this reduces their individual autonomy and thus their professional standing. He also asserts that, while nursing is striving to develop a unique body of knowledge, this detracts from patients possessing knowledge and disempowers them. He suggests that focusing on developing the body of nursing knowledge is for the benefit of nurses rather than for the patient and, as such, detracts from the service ideal. He further asserts that there is an alternative route to gaining professional status and that is through clinical professionalism that is independent of medical supervision. This issue will be revisited later in this chapter in the discussion relating to expanding roles.

So far, it has been argued that, on a superficial level, nursing meets the criteria for being a profession, but on closer inspection it falls down on several counts. Leddy and Pepper (1998) therefore suggest that nursing should more accurately be considered as an emerging profession. Alternatively, it could be argued that the pursuit of traditional professional status is wholly misplaced and that nursing would be better suited to redefining professionalism. Davies (1996) argues that the struggle to gain mastery over knowledge is an outmoded masculine trait of the traditional professions. She suggests that the concept of knowledge as the source of power needs to be re-examined in the light of changing societal expectations and contemporary health care. Her vision is for 'new professionalism', which incorporates reflective practice, shared decision-making and supported practice. Walsh (2000) also suggests that the generally accepted criteria for a profession have little relevance today and that all health-care workers should be looking at empowering patients; sharing knowledge and working across traditional boundaries in the spirit of interprofessional collaboration and user involvement. He contends that reversing the concern with professional status will return nursing to a greater service ideal and a greater focus on the needs of the patient, rather than the needs of nurses.

In summary, there are well-established criteria within sociological texts to help measure whether an occupational group has reached professional status. Nevertheless, there is continued debate as to whether nursing meets these criteria. Additionally, the functionalist approach to professionalism has its own critics and there is an emerging call for nursing to refocus its attention on the needs of the patient rather than its preoccupation with attaining professional status.

Activity 6.2

Irrespective of whether you believe that nursing is a profession or not, the NMC has a
clear expectation that nurses will act in a professional manner. A nurse's personal
values will characterise their professional practice.
Spend a few minutes considering what you consider to be professional practice and list
the main concepts that you believe underpin it.

You may have thought of professional practice being related to giving
the best possible care; treating people with respect; being able to explain
the reasons for your actions, and working with others in a collaborative
manner. These are all important but perhaps the most important concept in
relation to a nurse pursuing professional practice is that of accountability
(NMC 2002). There are many complex and circular arguments related to
trying to define accountability. Perhaps the most noteworthy are those discussions that attempt to unravel the connections between accountability
and the related concepts of responsibility, authority and autonomy. These
concepts will now be discussed and their interrelationships explored.

THE PRECONDITIONS LEADING TO ACCOUNTABILITY

According to the NMC (2002, 3), accountability means 'that you are
answerable for your actions and omissions, regardless of advice or directions from another professional'. Thus, nurses must be able to defend their
actions and explain the rationale for these based upon up-to-date knowledge, sound clinical decision-making and a knowledge of the patient's
wishes. It is not sufficient to act on another's orders unquestioningly or
hide behind a cloak of ignorance. For example, a junior staff nurse who
gives unprescribed medication on the orders of a more experienced staff
nurse would be held accountable for his or her own practice.

Nonetheless, seeking advice from specialist colleagues who have the
appropriate knowledge and authority would be the correct course of action
on many occasions, as part of the problem-solving process in clinical practice. For example, seeking the advice of a physiotherapist in relation to
rehabilitation exercises for a patient. Thus, the basis for accountability lies
in the nurse's competence to practise and in their conduct when practising.
Prior to the 1992 version of the Code of Professional Conduct (UKCC
1992a), the issue of accountability was not clearly articulated as a professional expectation, the inherited values of duty and responsibility being the
normal expectations at that time.

In today's health-care arena, the nurse is not only accountable to the
NMC as the regulatory body, but also to their employer in relation to
employment law, and to the patient and the public at large in relation to
civil law and the duty of care. However, in order to be held accountable,
there are some preconditions that need to be met. Bergman (1981) suggests

that these are ability, responsibility and authority. Moreover, Batey and Lewis (1982a) maintain that autonomy should also be added to these preconditions for accountability (see Fig. 6.1).

COMPETENCE

The ability of nurses to carry out their role competently is dependent upon them having sufficient knowledge and skill to fulfil the requirements of that role. The regulatory body for nursing and midwifery has the responsibility for ensuring that educational programmes that lead to initial registration and post-registration qualifications produce nurses who are fit for practice. However, it is the registered nurses' responsibility to maintain their professional knowledge and competence (NMC 2002). Thus, there is both collective and individual responsibility within nursing to ensure that the workforce has the ability to carry out its work in a competent manner.

RESPONSIBILITY

Responsibility 'is a charge for which one is answerable' (Batey & Lewis 1982a,14) and, as such, nurses accept responsibility as part of their role for interventions that fall within the accepted domain of nursing. The nursing interventions that are accepted as falling within the scope of nursing are taught within pre-registration courses so that, on registration, nurses can

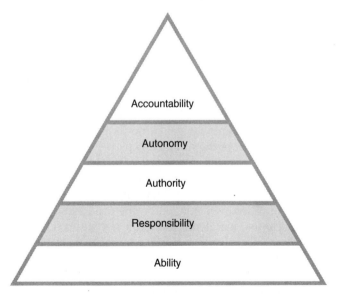

Figure 6.1 Model of preconditions leading to acccountability. (After Bergman 1981, with permission of the International Council of Nurses.)

accept full responsibility for implementing these. During educational pro-grammes, the responsibility for many nursing interventions is delegated to students so that they have some experience of carrying them out under supervision. Thus, although a student may accept the responsibility for car-rying out a nursing intervention, such as wound care, it is the nurse super-vising them who is professionally accountable for the outcome. The supervising nurse should, therefore, think carefully about whether it is appropriate to delegate the task to another and also be prepared to super-vise the activity. For example, if the student has had sessions on wound healing, a demonstration of aseptic technique in the skills laboratory and has a clear understanding of infection control procedures, then it would be reasonable to assume that they had sufficient ability and could accept responsibility for tending to a patient's wound care under direct supervi-sion. While the student cannot be held professionally accountable, in accepting the charge for a task they are answerable to the patient for carry-ing it out in a proficient manner. They are also answerable to their supervisor and employer in following guidance offered and alerting them to any problems that may arise.

In addition to responsibilities that come from within the discipline of nursing itself, there may also be responsibilities that are assigned from external sources such as the employer. An example may be additional roles deemed by the employer to be appropriate for nurses to carry out. These are often duties that are covered in hospitals when those who usually carry them out are off duty. For example, ward nurses may be delegated the role of being bed manager at the weekend. These will be discussed in more detail in the section on expanding nursing practice.

AUTHORITY

In order to carry out their responsibilities legitimately, nurses also require the authority to do so. The authority vested in nurses comes from a variety of sources that Batey and Lewis (1982a) cite as being the authority of the situa-tion, authority of expert knowledge, authority of position and authority of the group. The authority of the situation is usually related to emergency sit-uations, where nurses may take on roles they might not usually adopt owing to the nature of the emergency, for example, in a major incident scenario. The authority of expert knowledge links very much to the specialist education that is required in order to be entered on the professional register. The fact that a registered nurse has demonstrated a minimum level of knowledge vests them with the licence to practise and, as such, gives them the authority to practise in a manner set out by their regulatory body and employer.

Thus, the registered nurse has the legitimate power to carry out those nursing duties required in their everyday work. In some cases, nurses may have continued their education and have attained expert knowledge and skills in a particular specialist area, for example a tissue-viability clinical nurse specialist. Such nurses then have additional authority tied to their position. This authority should be clear in their role or job description. For example, it would be clear in the role description of a clinical nurse specialist that they have the authority to advise others on appropriate wound-care products or support surfaces for the prevention of pressure ulcers. The clinical grading system in the NHS also confers differential authority on different grades of nurses. For example, the D grade staff nurse's role description would differ significantly from a G grade ward manager's role and the authority invested in those roles would reflect this. Thus, while both a D grade staff nurse and a G grade ward manager are both professionally accountable, they would have different levels of organisational accountability dependent upon the level of authority invested in their respective roles. The final type of authority, that of authority of the group, is the authority vested in a formally constituted group by dint of the membership's expert knowledge and position. A good example of this type of authority would be a group set up to validate standards or protocols within a directorate. The group's authorisation is required before the policies or protocols can be adopted within the directorate.

AUTONOMY

So far, the discussion on the preconditions for accountable practice and, thus, professional practice have been fairly straightforward. A nurse needs to have the ability or competence to carry out their role, take on the responsibility of doing so and have the rightful authority to fulfil these responsibilities. Bergman (1981) would argue that, if all these conditions are met, then a nurse can be called to account for their actions. However, Batey and Lewis (1982b,13) contend that 'accountability is an exercise in futility and an experience in failure unless it is linked to nursing service's autonomy'. They argue that, as long as others have the power to veto a nurse's discretionary decisions, then they are not autonomous and so cannot be held accountable. Walsh (2000) concurs and states that nurses cannot be held accountable without being able to do what they think is right for the patient.

The question of autonomy in nursing practice is problematic. It is evident from the literature that the concept of autonomy is poorly understood and requires clarification (Ballou 1998, Wade 1999, Wilkinson 1997). While some authors seem to regard autonomy as synonymous with independence and a lack of control by external agents (Batey & Lewis 1982b), others recognise that it is not an all-or-nothing state and that there may be varying degrees of autonomous practice (Wade 1999, Wilkinson 1997). However, most literature agrees that autonomy in nursing practice is about the right to practise in line with the professional code or agenda.

As discussed in an earlier section, nursing practice can be limited by the medical profession; for example, at present, most nurses are dependent upon doctors to prescribe appropriate medication for patients or order relevant investigations. As such, nurses are not truly autonomous as some parts of their roles are dependent or interdependent. Wilkinson (1997) contends that to be truly independent is idealistic and undesirable. He suggests that it is more appropriate for nurses to be aware of what external factors control their practice and to challenge these when it affects their ability to care for their patients in the way they would wish. This links to the notion of ability being a prerequisite to accountability. If a nurse is able to make clinical decisions based on sound evidence and professional judgement, and can demonstrate this to those who have the power to veto their decisions, it is hoped that they would be able to persuade them that this is the right course of action.

MacDonald (2002) agrees and suggests that we should view nurses' and other health-care workers' autonomy as relational, as they are not only dependent on working in an institutional culture that is supportive of their capacity for independent judgement, but also upon supportive social relations. MacDonald expands upon this point by noting that, even though nursing and medicine are self-regulating, the privilege is granted by society and, thus, autonomy is only ever relational to the overall societal structure. Wade (1999) also points out that true professional autonomy is not realistic for any health-care profession, owing to the growing involvement of governmental agencies in the business of health care. This is as true for the medical profession as it is for nursing. For example, in the pursuit of evidence-based practice and the best use of scarce resources, the National Institute for Clinical Excellence develops and publishes guidelines that health-care professionals are expected to follow. Additionally, National Service Frameworks are setting the agenda for developments in several clinical specialities, which can limit the autonomy of those practising within those specialities.

The focal point for all these discussions, however, should be on what is in the best interests of the patient, rather than political shadow-boxing to prove who can win an argument. Wade points out that, in most discussions of autonomy, definitions do not take account of the centrality of the client. She claims that, to achieve positive outcomes for a client, health-care professionals should be engaged in collective enterprise and that autonomy involves 'affiliative relationships with clients and collegial relationships with others' (Wade 1999, 312). This suggests that nurses should be more concerned with doing the right thing for their patients than with arguing about who makes the final decisions. Thus, most nurses have autonomy relative to their position in the health-care organisation. This may be based on their expertise, experience or role, but should always be within the scope of nursing and exercised in the best interests of the patients they are caring for.

ACCOUNTABILITY

It has been shown that accountability is a complex concept and that certain preconditions are required before nurses can be accountable (see Fig. 6.1). However, these preconditions are sometimes absent and the nurse is left in a precarious position as far as accountability is concerned. For example, scarce resources may mean that a nurse is unable to provide the wound dressing that evidence suggests would aid optimum wound healing for a patient or they may not be consulted in essential end-of-life decisions about a patient in their care. These examples illustrate how difficult it can be for nurses to act in a manner which accords with their Code of Professional Conduct in everyday practice. Perhaps it is the nurses' conduct in striving for best practice and acting in their patients' best interests in everyday situations that truly reflects accountability in action.

Activity 6.3

Think about your own practice and list some of the issues that limit your ability to always act in your patients' best interests.

You may have noted lack of resources, lack of knowledge or the lack of authority to take a certain course of action. Often nurses feel that they are reliant on others to be able to carry out their role. For example, you may have to wait for a doctor to prescribe medication in order that you can effectively manage a patient's problem, or you may feel that the care your patient has received has been rather disjointed and that it would have been better for the patient to have dealt with fewer people. These issues are often linked to nurses expressing the desire to expand their sphere of practice so that they can improve the care their patient receives. The concepts of responsibility, authority, autonomy and accountability are very relevant to discussions of expanding roles as part of professional practice, and this issue will now be reviewed.

EXPANDING ROLES IN NURSING PRACTICE

As technology develops, the profile of the patient population changes and expectations of the health service increase, the role of nurses expands to meet the requirements of the patient and the changing health service. Historically, nurses carried out care that was considered to be menial and requiring a low level of knowledge and skill. However, as time has gone on, nurses have extended their roles. Initially, this extension of role was a direct response to taking on tasks that the medical teams deemed suitable for delegation.

In 1977, the Department of Health (DoH) issued guidance on extended roles as there were growing concerns that nurses were being asked to take on roles for which their pre-registration training had not prepared them (DoH 1977). The guidance clearly stated that nurses could only take on extended roles that had been delegated by doctors and that training had to be undertaken prior to undertaking extended roles. The training had to be approved by the nurse's employers and this spawned the issue of certificates of competence to undertake extended roles such as administering intravenous drugs. This practice of 'certificated extension' continued in a rather *ad hoc* fashion, but it became increasingly obvious that some nurses were required to extend their actual roles, rather than simply extending the repertoire of tasks that doctors had delegated to them.

In 1992, the UKCC offered guidance on this subject with the publication of 'The scope of professional practice' (UKCC 1992b). They acknowledged that pre-registration programmes are a foundation for professional practice and that continuing education is required as the demands of nursing practice expand. They declared that the practice of certificated extension detracted from the holistic nature of nursing practice and that, in future, as roles expanded, nurses themselves were to be responsible for ensuring that they were adequately prepared to undertake new roles. They further asserted that any expansion in role had to be primarily in the best interests of the patient, and should not compromise existing roles and responsibilities.

This declaration by the UKCC clearly set the agenda for role expansion, being a result of the need to improve services for patients rather than nurses simply taking on tasks that doctors no longer wished to undertake. For many nurses the publication of this document did little to change their everyday practice. Many employers still demanded certificates as proof of competence and the majority of nurses practised within the generally accepted sphere of nursing. However, for those nurses who were trailblazing new roles and expanding practice beyond that normally pursued by nurses, this opened up a whole new debate on levels of practice and the educational requirements needed to meet these.

Much research and literature in the last decade has been focused on attempts to quantify the nature of the differences between specialist and advanced practice, to delineate the differences between the multitude of new roles and to define the professional characteristics of nurses in these roles (e.g. see Dunn 1997, Finlay 2000, Hamric et al 1996, McGee et al 1996). The UKCC expressed a commitment to support the development of advanced practice, but finally concluded that it could not deliver a checklist of standards as this would conflict with the autonomous nature of many of the roles (UKCC 1997a) and would not fit with the edicts of 'The scope of professional practice'. The most recent Code of Professional Conduct (NMC 2002) replaces both the previous version of the code and the 'scope' document (UKCC 1992a, 1992b). It clearly expresses the need for nurses to maintain their professional knowledge and competence required for 'lawful, safe and effective practice without direct supervision' (NMC 2002, 8). It also states that, if an aspect of practice falls beyond the nurse's level of competence, then help and supervision must be sought until the nurse and the employer consider the requisite skills and knowledge have been attained.

PREPARATION FOR NEW ROLES

The NMC emphasise that each nurse is accountable for ensuring they are adequately prepared to undertake new roles but also note that the employer has a duty to ensure that any preparation is adequate. This links very clearly with the principles of clinical governance where the NHS organisations are accountable for improving quality and safeguarding standards (DoH 1998), and is timely in the light of research that highlighted that support from nurse managers and senior clinicians was vital to advancing nursing practice (Wilson-Barnett et al 2000).

There is a vast array of new roles where nurses have expanded their professional practice beyond the normally accepted sphere of nursing. For example, nurse practitioners operate in a variety of acute and primary care settings, and nurse consultants are being appointed in several clinical specialities. These may be indicative of what Porter (1992) classes as clinical professionalism, as nurses in many of these types of role do have a high level of autonomy and work without medical supervision. The interface between nurses in these roles and other health professionals has produced some innovative service developments, such as heart failure services, and are good examples of collaborative working across traditional professional boundaries. However, the real crux of the issue is that, above all, any new role must be for the good of the patient and enhance the quality of the service they receive.

Nurses in any role are accountable for their practice and must ensure that any role expansion meets this basic requirement. Thus, if a nurse finds that an emerging role change is merely for the convenience of the organisation, for instance reducing junior doctors' working hours, and detracts from other facets of their role, then they must resist and challenge the change. If, however, parts of their role can be delegated to others to accommodate their own role expansion, then this is acceptable, but only if it meets the best interests of the patient. Nurses need to be mindful of eroding their traditional focus on caring by delegating major parts of their work to others, such as health-care support workers. The major difficulty for most nurses when faced with clinical dilemmas such as these is how they can judge what is best for the patient both on an individual level and when looking at changes to service delivery to enhance quality of care, such as pre-admission clinics and other nurse-led initiatives. This relates to the earlier debate on whether nursing is a profession, where it was suggested that nurses might make better use of their time by redefining professionalism, rather than aspiring to attain an outmoded notion of it.

Perhaps in the same vein, nurses should stop focusing on trying to delineate varying levels of practice and whether they are autonomous within these roles, and instead work with other health-care professionals and patients to try to provide innovative and creative ways of improving services within the constraints of limited resources. Kenny (2002) contends that nursing should then be able to articulate its own unique contribution to health care within a framework of interprofessional collaboration, working across traditional boundaries for the benefit of patients. This would require a degree of refocusing for most health-care workers, not just nurses; but if nurses cannot demonstrate their own value to the team, there is the danger that they could be replaced with cheaper workers to the detriment of the patient.

SUMMARY

This chapter has explored the debate relating to whether nursing is or is not a profession, and it has been suggested that nurses need to explore new definitions and expressions of professionalism. The concept of accountability has been investigated in relation to the preconditions required for nurses to truly embrace it as part of their professional practice. The issues of competence, responsibility, authority and autonomy were discussed in relation to accountability in nursing. Finally, expanding roles for nurses have been discussed in relation to the changing health-care arena. Again, it has been suggested that the focus for professional nursing practice should be on deciding exactly what the unique contribution of the nurse is within the health-care team, rather than merely expanding their roles to suit organisational needs.

7

How do we make decisions about care?

INTRODUCTION

In the modern health-care arena, patients often have complex problems that require attention. Nurses, alongside their colleagues from other health-care disciplines, have to make decisions about the care they will deliver to these patients. How do nurses make decisions about care that are appropriate and effective? Do they utilise theory and research to inform the decisions they make? How do they choose which evidence will inform these decisions? In this chapter the methods used by nurses to make decisions in their everyday practice is considered. The nursing process as a problem-solving approach to nursing is reviewed and critiqued. The move towards using integrated care pathways (ICPs) is explored in the light of evidence-based interdisciplinary working. Finally, the range of skills required to make effective clinical decisions, and the evidence on which these are based, is examined.

INTENDED LEARNING OUTCOMES

By the end of this chapter you will:

1. be able to discuss the stages of the nursing process and the knowledge and skills required to carry these out competently

2. critically discuss the advantages and disadvantages of using the nursing process in nursing practice
3. appreciate the significance of integrated care pathways in the process of care delivery
4. begin to appreciate the range of clinical reasoning and decision-making skills required in contemporary nursing practice.

WHAT DECISIONS DO NURSES HAVE TO MAKE?

During their everyday practice, nurses are constantly required to make decisions about the care they provide for their patients. In order to make these decisions, nurses must be able to sift through the wealth of information that is available to them and make judgements that are based on sound reasoning skills. For nurses, learning to reason is just as important as learning about pathophysiology or fundamental nursing skills. The ability to think critically, make judgements and come to decisions based on the evidence available are skills that are imperative for the professionally accountable nurse. Critical thinking involves adopting a questioning approach and looking for a range of solutions to problems (Leddy & Pepper 1998).

Most experienced nurses have highly developed critical thinking skills that enable them to exercise a wide range of clinical reasoning and decision-making skills in their practice. Nurses with less expertise may not have developed such a range of skills, owing to lack of knowledge and experience. Nonetheless, they should be able to adopt a systematic approach to patient care in order to be able to give a rationale for their actions. Nurses have to develop their clinical reasoning and critical thinking skills over time, but are initially taught how to use a problem-solving approach to care delivery. The nursing process is the most commonly adopted approach to achieve this (Alfaro-LeFevre 1998). For the last 20 years, most nursing documentation in the UK has been based on the nursing process, comprising health assessment forms, individual care plans and evaluation sheets or progress notes. In the following sections, the nature of the nursing process is explored, and the advantages and disadvantages of using it are discussed.

WHAT IS THE NURSING PROCESS?

The nursing process is a problem-solving and decision-making tool that comprises five interrelated stages: assessment, nursing diagnosis, planning, implementation and evaluation (see Fig. 7.1). It provides a logical and systematic method of addressing problems and making decisions about the most appropriate and effective way to deliver care to individual patients. However, the stages of problem-solving are not unique to nursing and

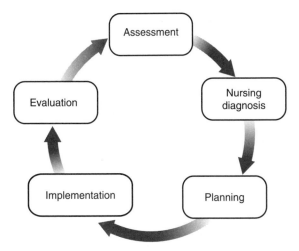

Figure 7.1 The nursing process.

Kataoka-Yahiro and Saylor (1994) propose that the nursing process is simply a discipline-specific version of critical thinking. Furthermore, Leddy and Pepper (1998) compare the steps of the nursing process with those of generic problem-solving and those of the scientific method. They note that others also use problem-solving in their everyday work. For example, an electrician will assess a piece of faulty equipment, diagnose the problem and discuss alternative means of repairing it. They will then plan how they can mend it, carry out the necessary repairs and then test the equipment to check that their work has been effective. It can be seen then, that the use of problem-solving and critical thinking are not the sole remit of the nurse, but the manner in which nurses utilise these in their everyday practice warrants further investigation if we are to understand how they develop their skills throughout their careers.

The nursing process was introduced to the UK in the late 1970s by the General Nursing Council (GNC) when it updated the pre-registration nursing syllabus. This was an attempt to improve the quality of patient care in a move away from task-centred and fragmented care towards a more holistic and individualised approach to care delivery. It was also later adopted by the United Kingdom Central Council for Nursing, Midwifery and Health Visiting (UKCC), which directed that student nurses should be required to demonstrate competence in assessing, planning, implementing and evaluating care as a prerequisite to registration (UKCC 1989).

Activity 7.1

Think about the stages of the nursing process.
Note what each stage entails, and describe the knowledge and skills the nurse requires
   to complete each stage successfully.

Assessment

In the assessment stage, the nurse systematically collects data about the patient's health status. This is a continuous process rather than a 'one-off' activity, and the subsequent stages of the nursing process are reliant upon an accurate and comprehensive assessment. The aim of the nursing assessment is to ascertain the patient's usual activities and how these have been altered, owing to their current ill-health episode, or how their lifestyle or family history may predispose them to particular health problems.

In order to carry out a comprehensive assessment, the nurse must collect and collate data about the patient from a variety of sources, including direct questioning, observation, clinical measurement and other health-care practitioners, such as paramedics or general practitioners. Once this has been done, data need to be validated and then organised into meaningful patterns. Validation of data is required so that errors are not made in problem identification. For example, if nurses suspect that an older patient is disorientated as a result of an acute confusional state, rather than a chronic dementia, they need to validate their assumptions by discussing the patient's usual cognitive abilities with their relatives to determine whether the confusion is a recent or long-term phenomenon. They also need to isolate factors that may precipitate an acute confusional state, such as a urinary tract infection, dehydration or constipation. This validation helps to avoid the nurse making assumptions or jumping to incorrect conclusions (Alfaro-LeFevre 1998).

While the nursing process clearly guides the nurse to assess their patient before making a diagnosis, it does not explain exactly *what* the nurse should assess. However, nursing models do articulate what the nurse needs to assess and the role of the nurse in health-care delivery. Thus, nurses also need to be taught about nursing models in order to use them in conjunction with the nursing process (see Ch. 3 for a discussion on nursing models).

Nursing diagnosis

The second stage of the nursing process is to identify patient problems that can be resolved, prevented or managed by appropriate nursing actions. This is termed making a nursing diagnosis. Unlike the medical diagnosis, which focuses on the disease state and pathophysiology of the patient, the nursing diagnosis focuses on the patient's symptoms. For example, a medical diagnosis may be that the patient has a chest infection. However, the nursing diagnosis would be related to the patient's symptoms of breathlessness and their resultant inability to carry out everyday activities.

The use of nursing diagnoses has taken two very different paths in the UK and the USA (Hardwick 1998). This can partly be explained by the reasons the nursing process was initially adopted in these countries. In the UK, the nursing process was adopted in an attempt to improve the quality of care the patients were receiving, yet in the USA its inception was more focused on establishing professional status and an attempt to develop a unique knowledge base for nursing (de la Cuesta 1983).

In the USA, nursing diagnoses have been organised into a nationally accepted hierarchy by the North American Nursing Diagnosis Association (NANDA). The wording and definitions of these diagnoses are validated and published by NANDA, and nurses utilise these validated diagnoses in their care-planning activities (Hogston 1997). Additionally, researchers have attempted to verify these diagnoses by testing their validity in the clinical setting and attempting to measure patient outcomes related to particular nursing diagnoses and their related nursing actions.

In the UK, nurses tend to identify each patient's problems or make nursing diagnoses on an individual basis, or utilise core or computerised care plans. Although some European countries, such as Sweden and Spain, have attempted to adopt the American taxonomy of nursing diagnoses, there is little consensus as to whether this should be implemented elsewhere (Hogston 1997). The recent employment of ICPs in the UK suggests that this will be unlikely in the future (see later sections for further discussions relating to ICPs).

Planning

The planning stage is directed toward negotiating appropriate goals with the patient and then determining the most effective means of achieving these. Goals help both the nurse and the patient to determine how the patient's problems will be addressed. Goals need to be developed with the patient's actual and potential abilities in mind, and should be prioritised. In other words, they need to be realistic and in priority order. At times, it may help both the nurse and the patient to plan care if the goals are divided into long-term and short-term goals.

It is important that goals are patient focused and couched in terms of what the patient, rather than the nurse, will be able to achieve. In order to aid evaluation, they should also be specific and measurable in some way. Once goals have been agreed, nurses then use their expertise to determine the most effective means for the patient to achieve the goals set. Once the nurse and patient have agreed the plan of care, the nurse needs to document this in the form of a care plan, which concisely delineates set goals in priority order, nursing actions and dates for review. This written plan will then guide all nurses who care for the patient.

Implementation

In this stage, the nurse is required to carry out the planned interventions in a skilled and timely manner. As the nursing process has an iterative structure, the nurse will constantly move backwards and forwards between stages. For example, if a patient's condition deteriorates or improves unexpectedly during the implementation stage, they will need to be reassessed, and the plan of care will need to be adjusted.

Evaluation

The evaluation of care is critical in order to ascertain whether patient problems have been resolved or whether the plan of care requires adjustment. The nurse and patient need to determine at preset times whether sufficient progress has been made towards achieving their goals at this stage (formative evaluation), or whether the goals have been achieved by the date set (summative evaluation). If a goal has been achieved then the problem has been resolved and no further intervention is required. However, if progress towards goal attainment is slower than predicted, the nurse needs to investigate why this has occurred and adjust goals or care accordingly.

KNOWLEDGE AND SKILLS USED IN THE NURSING PROCESS

The knowledge and skills required to employ the nursing process are numerous. Firstly, the nurse has to have the interpersonal skills to initiate and develop a therapeutic relationship with the patient in order to carry out the assessment. The nurse also requires expertise in communication skills to be able to elicit the information he or she requires in a sensitive and caring manner. An ability to use appropriate questioning techniques and to listen to the patient's responses, and then interpret these responses, is paramount.

Skills of critical analysis are also essential, as data must be organised into meaningful patterns to aid diagnosis. Nurses must be able to test out their initial diagnoses and then refine them. This parallels the hypothetico-deductive process of the scientific method. For example, a nurse may begin with general questions and then focus them to follow up on specific cues and validate tentative diagnoses or hypotheses.

The skills of identifying cues and relating these to their knowledge base, and also demonstrating an understanding and application of theories and principles, from both the natural and behavioural sciences, to the patient are required for a comprehensive assessment (Johnson & Webber 2001). Additionally, nurses must be able to record accurately and concisely their assessment so that other members of the health-care team can access the information. These skills are rarely fully developed in the junior nurse and, yet, it is interesting to note that it is often these very nurses who are asked to carry out the initial patient assessment and make nursing diagnoses. Registered nurses should be mindful of this when they are supervising more junior staff and delegating work. It is the registered nurse who is professionally accountable for ensuring that care is based on an accurate and comprehensive assessment, and they need to determine whether the junior nurse can do this without direct supervision (see Ch. 6 for a fuller discussion on accountability).

To make a nursing diagnosis, the nurse needs to have the ability to analyse all the information gathered during the assessment and make judgements as to what data are relevant and what is not relevant to the patient's current health problem. They have to recognise patterns and compare these to norms and theories, as they have to explain how the patient's symptoms relate to their underlying pathophysiology. It is understandable, then, that nurses with limited knowledge and experience may have difficulty in making the conceptual leap from the abstract to the particular, and may miss or ignore salient cues, owing to a knowledge deficit. For example, a junior nurse may note that a patient is breathless and, as a result of their limited experience, assume that this is due to a respiratory disorder. If a medical diagnosis is not yet available, they may miss other cues, such as swollen ankles or chest discomfort, which may indicate that the breathlessness is more likely to be of cardiac origin. This significantly impacts upon their ability to plan appropriate care successfully in the next stage.

At the planning stage, the nurse needs to draw on the previously mentioned skills of critical analysis, comprehension, application and explanation, but they also need the additional skill of being able to predict what interventions will produce the desired outcomes in a manner that is both effective in terms of resources and acceptable to the patient. For example, a nurse may have evidence that larval therapy is an effective method of debriding a wound, yet the patient may not consent to this form of treatment if they find it unpalatable, and the nurse needs to be aware of alternative methods.

To implement the planned care, the skills required relate mainly to the nurse's technical ability and psychomotor skills in performing nursing actions in a safe and effective manner. In terms of theoretical terminology, it is here that the nurse endeavours to influence and control phenomena in nursing. For example, they will attempt to maintain optimum conditions for psychological recovery or wound healing.

Evaluation necessitates all the previously discussed skills used in the first four stages of the nursing process. Additionally, nurses need to use their judgement to determine whether further nursing intervention is needed, whether referral to other agencies is appropriate or whether discharge is now required.

Activity 7.2

Review the previous sections, and think about what the benefits and criticisms of using the nursing process might be.

CRITIQUE OF THE NURSING PROCESS

The nursing process has been widely adopted and has been credited with being an excellent teaching aid for junior nurses in the development of their critical-thinking skills. It stresses the independent functions of the nurse and it is also thought to facilitate continuity of care through its documentation and language (Leddy & Pepper 1998). However, it is not without its critics.

While it is usually acknowledged that it is a valuable teaching tool for novice nurses, it has been noted that it is not consistent with the real world of nursing. Varcoe (1996) questions whether it captures what nurses do and suggests that, in reality, it may prescribe nursing as it should be rather than describe it as it actually is. For example, in theory, once the assessing nurse has documented the care plan, all nurses who care for the patient use it to guide their care. However, both O'Connell's (1998) and Waters' and Easton's (1999) research demonstrated that, in reality, nurses did not refer to care plans and their value was questioned by the nurses in the study. Taylor's (1997) research findings also noted that nurses rarely utilised documented care plans and that novice nurses were more likely to use role modelling in practice than to solve problems for themselves. While these were small studies and cannot be generalised, they do cast some doubt on whether the nursing process is used effectively in the real world of nursing. Additionally, the fact that its documentation is very time consuming may also militate against its effective use in the clinical arena despite Varcoe's (1996) contention that documentation is a consequence of implementation decisions rather than a requirement of the nursing process itself.

Lutzen and Tishelman (1996) suggest that, as the nursing process is seen to be a problem-solving approach, it unnecessarily biases nurses towards focusing on patient problems, rather than drawing on their strengths and resources. However, if used in conjunction with a nursing model that helps nurses to focus on health promotion, this bias can be balanced and the patient's resources can be utilised to prevent or manage health issues rather than simply viewing them as problems.

Varcoe (1996) also notes that nurses draw upon many sources of knowledge in their practice and that over-reliance on empirical data is inappropriate in nursing. Johnson and Webber (2001) concur with this viewpoint and contend that the nursing process is inappropriate for expert practice, as it is very biased toward the empiricist viewpoint and, thus, the legitimate use of nurses' intuitive grasp is minimised (see Ch. 2 for further discussion on this issue).

Varcoe (1996) also argues that, while the use of the nursing process has made what nurses do more visible, it has also decreased collaboration with other health-care workers in that the care plan is seen very much as the nurse's domain. This has not aided recent moves towards more collaborative practice and could have stifled the use of multidisciplinary patient records.

The positivist nature of the nursing process also maintains that nursing diagnoses are value free as they are derived from measurable and observable behaviour. However, Lutzen and Tishelman (1996) assert that nurses make value judgements when labelling patients with particular nursing diagnoses, and that the patients may not accept or recognise the diagnoses assigned to them. For example, if a nurse's and a patient's viewpoints clash, the nurse can label the patient as non-compliant. The patient may well have a clear rationale for their behaviour, which they would not construe as non-compliance, but common sense or a health-promoting activity. The balance of power can lead to the nurse's viewpoint being accepted as they are deemed to be the expert.

It can be seen that there are some valid criticisms of the nursing process and, although it can help inexperienced nurses to develop their problem-solving and critical-thinking skills, this is dependent upon adequate supervision and reflection upon the knowledge and skills required. Moreover, experienced nurses may not utilise it in their practice, and are likely to draw upon a wider repertoire of critical-thinking and reasoning skills than are required by the nursing process. These will be discussed further in other sections of this chapter.

Activity 7.3

Think about recent advances and initiatives in health care and reflect upon how they have influenced your capacity to deliver care to your patients.

Rapid advances in health care have affected every health-care worker in some way or another, and there are a multitude of topics that you may have thought about. It is likely that you will have considered advances in information technology and new treatments that have been developed as a result of research. As a nurse, the amount of new information available to you may, at times, seem overwhelming. You may also have thought about government initiatives, such as the call for increased collaboration between health professionals or the need to demonstrate the use of evidence-based practice. All of these issues have influenced the way care is delivered and have meant that many common practices are no longer appropriate.

As discussed in the previous section, the nursing process has been criticised for being time consuming and not facilitating collaboration with other health professionals. Some have noted that nurses can spend a considerable amount of time planning care and making decisions about patients on an individual basis, when, in reality, many patients with similar health problems require the same interventions (Walsh 1997). The use of standard or core care plans has to some extent reduced the amount of time nurses spend on care-planning activities, but has not really addressed the issue of increasing collaboration within the health-care team. The introduction of ICPs has partially addressed this issue, although they were originally introduced to demonstrate value for money to insurance companies, rather than to foster increased collaboration within the health-care team (Lowe 1998).

WHAT ARE INTEGRATED CARE PATHWAYS?

ICPs and clinical pathways, care maps and anticipated recovery paths are tools that are 'proactive, multidisciplinary designed, cost related, based on time frames and can be used as frameworks for the delivery of care and for concurrent and retrospective clinical audit' (Laxade & Hale 1995a, 290). They are based on the needs of particular groups of patients, sometimes referred to as diagnostic related groups, and are designed to ensure that a predetermined standard of care is coordinated and delivered within specified time frames (Arkell 1997). Thus, rather than members of the health-care team separately developing action plans on an individual basis for patients, the ICP is planned in advance by representatives from each discipline concerned, based on best practice that is derived from the available evidence.

The ICP clearly sets out what care a patient can expect within a given time frame and from whom, and also identifies any investigations, medications or teaching that the patient should receive. An ICP can cross sectoral boundaries, in that it can cover pre-admission to post-discharge, and can necessitate the involvement of primary, secondary and tertiary care. ICPs can also involve agencies outside of the health sector, such as social care. The ICP is then used as part or all of the patient's record of care (Johnson et al 2000). Any deviations from the pathway are recorded as variances (exception reporting) and this reduces the time needed for documentation, as only variances require documenting; routine care simply requires a signature. This meets the legal requirements for documenting care but reduces duplication. Variance analysis can inform improvements to the pathway and contribute to clinical audit. The pathway may be supplemented by the use of clinical guidelines or protocols. For example, an ICP designed for patients who have had a confirmed myocardial infarction will stipulate the investigations, treatment and care they should receive. The ICP is likely to include protocols derived from the National Service Framework for Coronary Heart Disease, such as referral for cardiac rehabilitation [Department of Health (DoH) 2000].

ICPs thus meet the government's agenda for quality (DoH 1998), in that they encapsulate clinical risk management, and allow standards to be predetermined and performance against set outcomes to be measured. The variance tracking facilitates continuous quality improvements, which sits well within the clinical governance agenda. Additionally, the mandatory multidisciplinary input clearly meets the government's requirement for increased collaboration between health-care professionals (DoH 1997).

Activity 7.4
Identify a group of patients that you have nursed, who required similar care. How might you go about developing a critical pathway for them and what difficulties do you think you might encounter in your endeavours?

DIFFICULTIES ASSOCIATED WITH ICPs

The major difficulty encountered with setting up ICPs is that of getting appropriate people to make time to meet and develop the ICP. Moreover, gaining consensus of what is best practice can be time consuming. It is important that this is recognised and that adequate resources are available for the release of appropriate staff. It has been suggested that an identified project leader is required, if momentum and motivation to complete the pathway is to be kept up (Johnson & Smith 2000).

It has also been reported that there has been resistance to the development of ICPs, as some health-care professionals believe that ICPs are inflexible, undermine their ability to exercise clinical judgment and do not meet individual patient needs (Lowe 1998). ICPs work best for patients when care and treatment is likely to follow a defined path; for example, elective surgery. It is important to note that ICPs will only ever be suitable for a certain percentage of the chosen diagnostic-related group. It is also impossible to devise ICPs for patients who have multiple pathologies, which run unpredictable courses, and these patients will continue to require individual plans of care. Therefore, it is imperative that patients are individually assessed to ascertain their suitability for the ICP. The reporting of variances, if expected outcomes are not met, also calls for the nurse or other health-care professional to judge what has caused the deviation from the pathway and make a decision as to the care or treatments necessary to put them back on track. Thus, clinical judgement and decision-making are an integral part of implementing ICPs. Additionally, as new evidence comes to light, ICPs need to be reviewed and updated.

The issue of accountability can also be problematic, if it is not clearly stipulated within the ICP who is responsible for implementing each part of the pathway, documenting it and acting upon variances. For example, if it is stipulated in the pathway that patients who undergo surgery require an X-ray on the first post-operative day, who ensures that this happens—the doctor, radiographer or nurse? This problem can be overcome in part by advances in technology. The development of electronic ICPs with integrated systems can set up automatic requests, for example for X-rays, once a patient is on the pathway (Norris & Briggs 1999). The issue of clinical governance is also pertinent in this respect, as it calls for an emphasis upon individual accountability, and for the organisation to set up clear lines of responsibility and accountability. Evaluations of ICP projects have indicated that these issues have been problematic (de Luc 2000, Johnson et al 2000). However, these studies also demonstrated positive outcomes in other areas, such as decreased length of stay for patients.

The whole issue of whether the effectiveness of ICPs has been demonstrated is a controversial one. There is a paucity of rigorous research in this area and many projects have not considered success criteria to aid this (Johnson & Smith 2000). Additionally, the reasons for developing an ICP have a bearing on whether they are deemed to be successful. De Luc (2000) gives the example that, if an ICP had been developed to maintain quality indicators at a lower cost, then a result that showed no adverse effect on quality would be a positive result. If, however, the ICP had been developed to improve quality, the same result would be viewed as negative. There remain many questions to be answered in this area, but the use of ICPs is being heralded by many as a new way of working that improves outcomes for patients and staff satisfaction, especially when used in a case management system (see Ch. 8 for further discussion on case management). They are not, however, the panacea for all patient care, and nurses still require sound reasoning and clinical decision-making skills to perform competently in the clinical arena.

Activity 7.5

Imagine that a patient that you are caring for suddenly develops chest pain. They state that this is the first time that they have experienced a pain as severe as this. You have to make a decision as to what to do next. Think about *how* you make that decision and the process you go through to determine what action to take.

DECISION-MAKING IN NURSING

Your clinical experience and the clinical area in which you are working will obviously influence the decisions that you make. If you are a student nurse, your course of action may be to alert a more senior member of staff to the patient's situation. If you are a qualified nurse, you may decide to contact a member of the medical team or you may decide to assess the nature of the pain before doing so. If you have experience in the cardiac field, you might decide to record a 12-lead ECG before contacting a doctor. However, you will have gone through a process of thinking in order to make a judgement and reach your decision. For example, the student nurse considered that chest pain could be a serious threat to the patient (judgement) and thus called for help from a more experienced colleague (decision). If the student had not perceived such a threat, they would probably have continued to care for the patient without consulting anyone else. In other words, nurses use their reasoning skills to make judgements and then choose between alternatives to make a decision.

In the following sections, some clinical decision-making models will be considered. However, before these are discussed, the concepts of critical thinking, clinical reasoning and clinical judgements will be delineated. While some authors contend that these terms can be used interchangeably (Thompson 1999), there are some who are quite explicit about the subtle nuances and differences between them (Johnson & Webber 2001).

CLINICAL REASONING AND CRITICAL THINKING

Clinical reasoning is 'the process of determining the existence and nature of a relationship between two or more concepts' (Johnson & Webber 2001, 53). Its importance in nursing is that the use of clinical reasoning enables nurses to use knowledge to answer questions, solve problems, predict outcomes and influence or control situations. Daly (1998) notes that there is a lack of consensus in the literature about what constitutes critical thinking. Brookfield (1987) (cited in Boychuk Duchscher 1999) suggests that critical thinkers identify and challenge assumptions; recognise the importance of context; explore and imagine alternatives, and engage in reflective scepticism in their search for new meanings. Moreover, Johnson and Webber (2001) state that critical thinking is often used interchangeably with the term 'reasoning', but they contend that critical thinking is the foundation for, rather than being the same as, reasoning. They suggest that a nurse might think critically and identify propositions, using both inductive and deductive approaches (see Ch. 1) without understanding the complexity of their nature and their significance.

Let us return to our patient with chest pain, who has a medical diagnosis of aortic stenosis. An inexperienced nurse may know that a patient with aortic stenosis might have chest pain as one of their symptoms and should be able to use their critical-thinking skills to outline the pathophysiology behind this phenomenon. Based on their experience of patients with chest pain being prescribed vasodilator drugs, they may ask why the patient has not been prescribed glyceryl trinitrate to alleviate their symptoms. A more experienced nurse would be able to explain that, although the chest pain is ischaemic in nature, that is, due to reduced blood flow, the prescription of vasodilators, in this instance, is inappropriate, as the reduced blood flow is due to obstruction of the valve, rather than narrowing of the coronary arteries. The experienced nurse has used their wider knowledge base, understanding of the context, experience and clinical reasoning to explain the situation, and can predict that administration of nitrates would, in fact, exacerbate rather than alleviate the symptoms in this instance.

Johnson and Webber (2001) further propose that critical thinking and reasoning are differentiated in that, although both use deliberate scientific thinking, reasoning also integrates more phenomenological thought. They contend that inexperienced nurses rely primarily on critical thinking and that, as they move towards expert practice, the phenomenological aspects of nursing, such as experiential knowledge and intuition, begin to be used. Experienced nurses also have the ability to reason abductively, that is, they have the ability to make 'a conceptual leap based on observations, experience, beliefs, and patterns to arrive at an educated guess about a phenomenon' (Johnson & Webber 2001, 61). Unlike novice nurses, they are able to move away from rule-bound actions to those that encompass a much more holistic approach. In summary, then, nurses move from the novice information-gathering stage to critical thinking and then develop clinical reasoning skills in their progression toward expert practice.

CLINICAL JUDGEMENT

Judgement is defined as the 'assessment of alternatives' (Thompson & Dowding 2002, 15). Cioffi (2002) emphasises the fact that effective nursing care is dependent upon good clinical decision-making, which in turn is based on accurate judgements. She maintains that nurses can improve the clinical judgements they make, if they have an understanding of the processes involved and what factors influence them.

Cioffi (2002) has reviewed pertinent judgement research, and notes that both experience and expertise can affect the way in which nurses make judgements. She summarises this by noting that individuals who have more clinical experience are often more accurate and that tasks with restricted amounts of information are linked to higher accuracy. Nurses seem to use past experiences when processing information, and Cioffi (2002) suggests that nurses with greater experience are thus able to utilise more heuristics, that is, 'rules of thumb' or short cuts. They have had repeated exposure to similar events (representativeness heuristic) and memories of particularly vivid or relevant cases (availability heuristic) to aid them in forming judgements. They are also more able to identify what is and is not relevant information. Less experienced nurses have a tendency to use mainly propositional knowledge. As a result, they can bias their judgements by an over-reliance on confirming information and an underestimation of disconfirming information; that is, they often ignore information that does not 'fit' with their tentative diagnosis of a situation.

In order to develop judgement skills, Cioffi (2002) recommends that nurses use strategies such as looking for what does not fit rather than what does. They should try to be specific when estimating probabilities, such as risk of falls, to consider reasons why a judgement may be incorrect and to respect ambiguity in information by remaining open.

CLINICAL DECISION-MAKING THEORIES

In order to make clinical decisions, nurses need to deal with complex information or data that can be qualitative or quantitative in nature and can often be conflicting. Not every nurse faced with the same information would make the same decisions. In order to understand how nurses and other health-care workers make decisions, it would be useful to consider some of the decision-making theories that have been put forward. These theories are usually either descriptive or prescriptive, that is, they either attempt to describe how decisions are made or they try to improve decision-making.

Information processing, or the hypothetico-deductive approach, is perhaps the most influential and well-known descriptive theory. This theory postulates that problem-solving can be analysed as two processes occurring at the same time. These two processes are 'understanding' and 'search'. The understanding process notes the stimulus that poses a problem and the search process is driven by that understanding (Taylor 2000). The stimulus information in the short-term memory 'unlocks' factual knowledge stored in the long-term memory. Thus, the nurse or other health-care worker encounters a patient or situation that stimulates memory-based cues and they then make tentative hypotheses about the situation. These are then interpreted to confirm or refute the initial hypothesis. In the final evaluatory stage, the nurse weighs up the alternatives and chooses the one favoured by the preponderance of evidence (Thompson 1999).

To illustrate, suppose a patient develops an unexplained pyrexia. The cue of 'high temperature of unknown origin' would 'unlock' several potential causes that could be investigated by the nurse and these could be pursued by the gathering of other evidence to confirm or refute the hypotheses.

The information processing theory sits within the systematic-positivist paradigm, and is one that has prompted much debate and research. However, proponents of a more intuitive–humanist paradigm suggest that there are other theories that more readily explain the way in which nurses make decisions. Perhaps the most influential proponent of this domain in nursing is Benner (1984). The basis of her theoretical viewpoint is that expert nurses do not rely on analytical principles to link their understanding of a situation to some form of action. For example, an experienced nurse may report that a patient needs to be closely observed because they feel that they are 'not right', without being able to identify any tangible clinical signs of a deteriorating condition other than a gut feeling that something is wrong. Rather, their clinical decisions are the result of an almost unconscious level of cognition or intuitive grasp of the situation. (See Ch. 2 for a fuller discussion of Benner's work.)

So which of these two standpoints most reflects real life and decisions made in the clinical situation? Thompson and Dowding (2002) suggest that these two approaches, although conceptually distinct, are two poles on a cognitive continuum and that, in real life, clinicians use a mixture of decision-making models. They contend that this viewpoint lends itself to further theoretical development and research, as findings in this field have so far been contradictory or inconclusive.

Prescriptive theories identify theoretically how an individual should make a decision. They are usually based on probability estimates of diagnostic fit. Perhaps the most influential theory in this area is Bayesian theory. Bayes' theorem is a statistical model that shows the way that new information leads to revision of judgements (Taylor 2000). While the use of Bayes' theorem may help researchers to investigate exactly how clinicians weigh up evidence, it does not take account of the context in which nurses work. Nurses rarely have to make decisions that are based on clear-cut criteria. One decision is often dependent upon another, or a patient may have multiple health problems that may militate against certain actions being taken. For example, a nurse may be able to predict the probability that a patient will develop a pressure ulcer on their sacrum, if they do not change their position or use a pressure-relieving mattress. However, if the patient is critically ill and has an unstable spine due to trauma and has an unstable cardiac arrhythmia, then these usual practices may cause more problems than they might solve. The nurse, in this instance, has to undertake a risk assessment of the benefits of initiating certain nursing care against the risks that this action might pose to the patient.

Both descriptive and prescriptive theories have helped us to understand some of the ways in which nurses make decisions but, perhaps more importantly, they provide theoretical frameworks on which to base research into this fascinating area. If we can better understand how clinicians make decisions and what influences them, then ways in which to improve decision-making skills may be discovered.

Activity 7.6

Think about the types of decisions that you have to make in your everyday practice. What tools are available to help you make those decisions and plan appropriate care?

AIDS TO DECISION-MAKING AND CARE PLANNING

We have already discussed the use of ICPs to aid the multiprofessional team in caring for clients in a manner that reflects both consistency and evidence-based practice. There are also other tools available to health-care workers to enhance their practice and to avoid having to spend time weighing up the preponderance of evidence when making decisions about the same things. Perhaps the most common of these tools in contemporary practice are clinical protocols or guidelines. Unlike ICPs, which cover a whole episode of care, clinical guidelines or protocols usually cover only one aspect of care. Examples include a protocol for removing intercostal drains and clinical guidelines relating to when and how to refer patients to specialist services. The aim of these clinical guidelines is to reduce inappropriate variability in care and to improve patient outcomes.

Clinical guidelines may be developed locally by specialist teams or nationally by professional organisations or government bodies. For example, the National Institute for Clinical Excellence (NICE) publishes guidelines at a national level and it is expected that these will be implemented locally. The strongest evidence that these guidelines can be based on is considered to be meta-analysis of randomised control trials, and the weakest is that from expert committee reports or clinical experience of respected authorities. Nevertheless, guidelines should always be based on the best evidence available, and government or professional bodies usually have access to this and the expertise to be able to evaluate its worth for the population under consideration. If clinical guidelines are required on a particular issue within your clinical area, it is well worth doing on-line searches of professional body or governmental web sites to determine if clinical guidelines already exist which you could adopt. Published guidelines should make reference to the evidence on which they are based, so that you can check that they are based on contemporary evidence.

Computerised decision support is also being developed in the NHS to aid decision-making. For example, NHS Direct is a 24-hour nurse-led advice service available that is supported by a computer-based decision-support programme. NHS Direct aims to help the public make decisions about their health. For example, they may phone to enquire whether a health problem necessitates a visit to the accident and emergency department or whether it can safely wait for a routine appointment to their general practitioner.

SUMMARY

In this chapter, some of the methods by which nurses and other health-care professionals make decisions about care have been explored and their usefulness outlined. Tools to aid decision-making have also been discussed.

Nurses use a variety of different types of information and skills to make decisions in their practice. Understanding the manner in which information is sought, appraised and processed gives some indication of how nurses can be helped to develop the requisite skills for sound decision-making. If nurses are to be truly accountable, their decisions need to be transparent and open to scrutiny. It is hoped that exploring these issues has raised awareness of the importance of being able to justify not only your decisions, but also the methods by which you have reached those decisions.

8

How do we manage care?

INTRODUCTION

Professional care does not just happen, it requires careful planning and, in the previous chapter, the way in which individual nurses make decisions about care was considered. In this chapter, the wider care arena is examined and the manner in which nurses organise care delivery is investigated. Individual nurses may prioritise their own workload, but care must be managed in such a way as to ensure coordination of services and continuity for the patient. No clinical area, whether it is primary, secondary or tertiary care, works in isolation and nurses are not the only health-care workers who provide care. Any organisation needs to bring staff together, such as nurses, doctors, allied health professionals and ancillary workers. This chapter explores task and patient allocation, team nursing, primary nursing and case management. Some of the factors that have influenced these systems of care delivery are examined and related to the concept of the named nurse. The development of new roles for nurses aimed at improving the management and delivery of care are briefly explored. In the light of recent government initiatives, the wider context of organisation of care is reviewed and clinical governance is outlined.

INTENDED LEARNING OUTCOMES

By the end of this chapter you will:

1. be able to discuss critically the relative merits and disadvantages of a number of care delivery systems

2. appreciate how the role of the nurse in different care delivery systems has been influenced by social and political factors
3. appreciate the factors that have influenced the emergence of new roles for nurses, and the implications these have for cross-boundary and interprofessional working
4. understand the concept of clinical governance, factors that have influenced its emergence in health care and outline the nurse's responsibilities within it.

Activity 8.1

Think about how care is organised in your clinical area and who makes decisions about patient care.
Think about the main advantages and disadvantages of this system.

You will probably have named a care delivery system, which has been agreed and developed by the nursing staff working in your clinical area and which best meets the needs of the speciality and fits with the available skill mix. Historically, the way in which care has been organised in nursing has been influenced by the social and political pressures of the era, and reflects the values of society about health and health-care provision. For example, when no hospitals or health-care system existed, care was managed in the patient's home by carers with no formal education. These carers either followed physician's orders, if they had the money to engage a physician, or relied on home remedies, if they could not. In the next section, care delivery systems that have been used in hospitals are discussed in the light of the context in which they were adopted. The impact this has had on both the nurse and patient care is examined, and the emergence of new roles for nursing is explored.

TASK ALLOCATION

This is the traditional, hierarchical system of care delivery that is sometimes referred to as functional nursing (Leddy & Pepper 1998). Task allocation was instituted when nursing was first emerging as a discipline and reflected its subservience to medicine (see Chs 1 and 2 for a fuller discussion of the emergence of nursing). A hierarchical chain of command was evident, whereby the ward sister/charge nurse decided what nursing care patients required in the light of the doctor's prescribed treatment. The work of the ward was then divided into a series of tasks and was delegated according to the complexity of the task. Experienced nurses were given the technical tasks, and junior nurses were delegated tasks considered to be basic and requiring less skill. The tasks tended to be focused on medical/technical aspects of care, rather than on human/interpersonal aspects

(Adams et al 1998). For example, a junior student might be delegated the patient washes, a senior student the simple dressings, and a staff nurse the drug administration and more complex dressings. Patients were, therefore, cared for by several nurses, who completed their assigned task and then moved on to the next patient.

In this method, efficiency was considered more important than continuity of care or patients' total needs. The ward sister/charge nurse retained control of the workload, made decisions about any changes in nursing care, communicated with other health-care professionals and was accountable for the care delivered within the ward. The Audit Commission (1991) reported that the ward sister/charge nurse seemed to know everything about every patient, while junior staff knew very little. Patients had little say in decisions about their care, which was delivered in a fragmented manner. This mode of working has been compared to a factory assembly line (Pontin 1999). Nurses accepted their delegated tasks and reported on their progress to the ward sister/charge nurse, but had no authority to make any changes to care. Task allocation reflected both society's view of nursing, and the nature of 'women's work' and the relative lack of power vested in the patient. The tasks tended to be focused upon physical care and very little attention was paid to the patient's psychological, cultural or social needs. In this mode of organisation, nurses were able to maintain a psychological distance from the patients. The nurse–patient relationship was limited to brief encounters with a series of nurses, rather than the development of meaningful and therapeutic relationships.

PATIENT ALLOCATION

Task allocation remained the dominant mode of care delivery within hospitals in the UK until the 1970s, although some literature suggests that it still persists in some quarters today, especially in times of staff shortage (Hilton & Goddard 1996). However, in the 1970s there was a general ideological shift in the NHS towards more patient-centred care (Adams et al 1998) and patient allocation was adopted as a new way of working. A general dissatisfaction with task allocation amongst qualified nurses and the perceived need to improve quality of care for patients strongly influenced this development. The General Nursing Council (GNC) introduced the nursing process in the 1970s in the UK (see Ch. 7 for a discussion on the nursing process) and the practice of task allocation did not fit with the requirements of individualised care.

Patient allocation meant that one nurse was allocated to care for several patients for a shift, rather than perform the same task for several patients. Thus, one nurse was able to plan and deliver total patient care for their allocated patients on that shift. They were able to use the nursing process to develop a plan of care, which was then documented and used as a template for other nurses who were allocated to that patient on subsequent shifts. However, Adams et al (1998) claim that the power base remained firmly with the ward sister and, although the focus shifted away from tasks towards patient need, continuity of care remained an issue, as nurses were often allocated different patients on consecutive shifts. Thus, the issue of shared responsibility remained and the ward sister/charge nurse was still deemed to be accountable for the care on the ward.

TEAM NURSING

Team nursing can be distinguished from patient allocation in that nurses and support workers are grouped together in a team and allocated patients for a certain time period (Gill et al 2000). The time period of allocation is variable, but nurses are generally allocated to teams for months rather than days. The team has a designated leader, who facilitates the sharing of expertise and coordinates care delivery as appropriate. This is deemed to be a less hierarchical structure than patient allocation. It is based on the assumption that nurses working together in a supportive team with varied expertise will be able to provide better care than an individual nurse and that nurses will gain greater job satisfaction (Adams et al 1998). Although there is a team leader, registered nurses are accountable for their own practice.

The advantages of team nursing are claimed to be improved continuity of care for patients; improved opportunity for the development of leadership skills in nurses, and closer supervision of junior and untrained staff. Nevertheless, although theoretically the setting up of teams appears straightforward, there are inherent difficulties in any organisational change and issues, such as managing off duty rotas, annual leave and attempting to change the ethos of 'getting the work done', can be complex and fraught with difficulties (Binnie 2000a, 2000b). Additionally, although there are many reported benefits of team nursing, there is limited empirical evidence to support these claims (Gill et al 2000). While it is acknowledged that team nursing can lead to a flatter hierarchy, with teams being responsible for communication with other health-care professionals and organising the patient's discharge, it can lead to complex lines of communication. For example, a medical team may have patients in several different teams and would need to liaise with a different group of nurses to discuss care for each patient. Binnie (2000c) discusses some of the difficulties this can pose, and highlights the need for lines of communication to be made explicit to all involved, with clear lines of accountability and responsibility agreed when implementing team nursing. Team nursing is often used as a stepping stone to the implementation of primary nursing, which takes further steps towards individualised and holistic care.

PRIMARY NURSING

This system of care delivery involves patients being allocated to an individual nurse rather than a team and the primary nurse having 24-hour responsibility for the patient from admission until discharge. In the absence of the primary nurse, associate nurses carry out the plan of care devised by the primary nurse. The main protagonist of this method of care delivery outlines the key concepts of primary nursing as being responsibility; continuity of care; direct communication, and care giver as care planner (Manthey 1992). While this mode of care delivery was popular in the USA from the 1970s, it was not implemented in the UK until the 1980s and then mainly by nursing development units (NDUs), such as the Burford and Oxford NDUs, which were set up to emphasise the therapeutic role of nursing (Ersser & Tutton 1991, Pearson 1988).

Primary nursing is seen as a vehicle for promoting continuity of care and patient participation in decision-making. Accountability for care is vested clearly with the primary nurse. This structure emphasises a collegial support structure and the role of the ward sister/charge nurse is consultant, educator and resource (Adams et al 1998).

Primary nursing can only be implemented if there are sufficient qualified staff in an area who have the requisite skills and experience to take on the role of primary nurse, and this has proved problematic in some areas. Additionally, there does not seem to be a consensus in the literature about whether primary nursing is actually a care delivery system or a philosophy, or both, and thus the mode of implementation varies enormously (Pontin 1999). The implications for this have been that much of the research that is said to evaluate the effectiveness of primary nursing cannot be compared, owing to variations in operational definitions.

Activity 8.2

How do these different care delivery systems fit with the concept of the named nurse? How do you implement the named nurse in your clinical area?

The development of team and primary nursing in the 1980s took place in the UK at the same time as a shift in emphasis in the health-care culture and ethos. There was a move towards viewing the patient as a consumer within a market-led health service (Steven 1999). The government of the time had already voiced its support for primary nursing as an ideal mode of care delivery and, in 1991, published the Patient's Charter, which introduced the concept of the named nurse.

THE NAMED NURSE

The Patient's Charter stated that patients could expect a named, qualified nurse to be responsible for their nursing care (Department of Health (DoH) 1991) and that this system would begin to be implemented by April 1992. This top-down approach to the implementation of the named nurse, rather like the implementation of the nursing process, was met with some resistance. While most nurses embrace the notion of individualised and holistic care, there remains a lack of clarity about exactly how the named nurse initiative should be implemented and many nurses remain unclear as to the implications for their own accountability (Dooley 1999).

Issues of skill mix and a perceived lack of resources required for the implementation of the named nurse were exacerbated by a shortage of trained nurses in the NHS, which became evident in the 1990s. Additionally, many have begun to question the rigour of much of the research that claims to demonstrate the benefits of team and primary nursing, which are both seen as vehicles for implementing the named nurse (Steven 1999). Moreover, in a well-executed study by Adams et al (1998), it was found that very few acute wards in hospitals fitted the three main 'ideal-type' nursing systems outlined above. They noted that, while many wards had characteristics of the commonly described care delivery systems, none of the areas had all the attributes of these systems. This begs the question of whether the descriptions of team and primary nursing in the literature are prescriptions of how nursing ought to be, rather than as it is actually practiced. In light of this, it is interesting to note that in the recent publication 'Your guide to the NHS' (DoH 2001b), which effectively replaces the Patient's Charter, no mention is made of the named nurse. This perhaps reflects the more recent concerns with patient outcomes, rather than the process, and the blurring of professional boundaries in care giving.

Activity 8.3

Think about the implementation of multidisciplinary integrated care pathways. How might this affect the way in which care is organised?

As discussed in Chapter 7, a greater emphasis on collaborative working across disciplines and the agenda of implementing evidence-based practice has resulted in the widespread adoption of managed care and integrated care pathways. For those areas that implement ICPs, the majority of patients have the ICPs implemented and documented at ward level. Nurses who manage the care in relation to the ICP may be working in a team or primary nursing system, and are responsible for ensuring that the ICP is followed as far as nursing interventions are concerned. The limitations of this way of organising care is that a primary nurse or team nurse is only concerned with nursing care, and also the patient's journey does not necessarily rest in only one department. For example, many patients undergoing major surgery may move from theatres to intensive care and then back to a ward, and have three different teams or primary nurses caring for them. Likewise, a patient being admitted for investigations may move from a day-case ward to the radiography department and back again. For the majority of patients who meet the expected outcomes of an ICP, this does not pose a problem. However, for patients who have unexpected variances or who are at high risk of these, there is a need for someone to coordinate care and troubleshoot when problems arise. Additionally, although nurses at a ward level can record variances and take appropriate action in relation to individual patients, there is a need to analyse variances across the care pathway and resolve patterns in aggregate variances from expected outcomes or standards of care (Schriefer & Botter 2001). For example, early removal of drains in intensive care may result in wound problems but these might not show up until the patient is returned to the ward. A recurring pattern of variances needs to be analysed and possible causes investigated so that they can be rectified.

In some areas, the need for an individual to be accountable for resolving these issues has been recognised, and the role of the case or care manager has evolved. Initially, these roles were adopted in the USA to ensure the successful operation of the system and to contain costs where possible. In the UK, these roles have evolved as part of risk management and quality improvement systems. The case manager's role is to connect previously unconnected parts of the system to ensure the patient's smooth transition across departmental and sector boundaries, to analyse variances and investigate ways of reducing these and the risk of untoward incidents. This role can be taken on by any health-care worker but increasingly has been taken on by nurses (Laxade & Hale 1995b). The case manager can be a discrete role or case management functions may be incorporated into existing roles, such as clinical nurse specialist or senior nurse. As the case manager has responsibility for coordinating all aspects of the ICP, they need to be given the authority to do so and this must be recognised by all care givers. This can mean a significant change in traditional power relations, especially if nurses take on the role and have the authority to investigate and suggest changes to medical practice as part of their role.

Activity 8.4

Can you think of any other new roles that nurses have taken on in recent years that cross traditional boundaries?
Have they affected the way care is organised?

Health care is expanding and dynamic, and the NHS will be unable to meet the increasing demand for care without role and practice expansion.

There is a need to look at ways of continually reviewing practice and ensuring that resources are being used in an effective and efficient manner (DoH 1998). The recent establishment of nurse consultant posts have in many instances attempted to fill gaps in service and provide innovative ways of enhancing care delivery. Examples include nurse consultants leading outreach teams from intensive care (Coombs & Dillon 2002) and nurse consultants running heart failure clinics (Coady 2002). Other more established roles, such as nurse practitioners in primary care and accident and emergency departments, have for some time been at the junction of nursing, medicine and sometimes radiography (Walsh 2000).

In a project to evaluate new roles in practice, Scholes and Vaughan (2002) identified three types of role development: complementary roles, substitution roles and niche developments. Complementary roles were the most well established and were mainly found in cancer services, where roles had developed in parallel with developments in treatments and services. Substitution roles were ones set up to deliver a service normally carried out by doctors and niche roles were those developed to fill a gap in current service provision. In all roles they found there were interprofessional tensions, such as the questioning of authority to make decisions, the perception of deskilling of nurses at ward level and the constraints of working within protocols. They found that many of these tensions related to issues of control and that medical dominance, though often exercised in a covert way, was very evident in the development of new roles, whether it be in issues of supervision or in the drawing up of protocols. They suggest that, in many instances, with substitution roles there was not a blurring of traditional boundaries but that boundaries had simply been redrawn. However, postholders in complementary roles and niche developments had greater freedom in their practice, and it was found that experiential wisdom and professional maturity were critical to the success of these posts.

As nurses take on new roles at a variety of levels, they in turn need to face the dilemma of examining their own role and handing over aspects of care to others, such as health-care support workers. This cannot be done without a careful examination of what nursing really entails and ensuring that nurses retain the parts of their role that reflect the essence of nursing care. This has posed major challenges in the development of educational programmes that will prepare the workforce for the health-care system of the future. There has not been a consensus on what is considered nursing work and what aspects can be handed over to ancillary staff. The arguments often reflect the various stakeholders' perspectives. For example, a manager who wants to ensure that all patients have their essential hygiene needs met may employ health-care assistants to achieve this, but it reflects a very task-oriented perspective. It can be argued that qualified nurses should be employed, as they have the skills and expertise to carry out full nursing assessments and develop therapeutic relationships with patients at the same time as meeting patients' hygiene needs. However, the counter argument is that nurses do not have the time to retain their entire current role and expand their practice at the same time. Thus, issues of skill mix are inextricably linked to the discussion on what nurses should be doing, especially in light of the recruitment and retention problems noted in nursing since the 1990s.

It is evident that many of the new roles discussed have helped the government to meet its health agenda of developing new ways of working and providing a workforce with sufficient numbers and the requisite skills (DoH 1997, 1998). However, how they ultimately impact upon the quality of health care requires rigorous evaluation, especially in light of the ongoing debate about professional boundaries, competence and multiskilling within health care and the implications this has for professional education (Masterson 2002).

ORGANISATION WITHIN THE NHS

We have already explored some of the ways in which nursing care can be organised, but this cannot be seen in isolation from how the health service is managed as a whole. In recent years, the concept of clinical governance has been introduced into the health service and it is to this that we will now turn our attention. The recent health-care agenda has moved towards challenging all clinical professionals to achieve excellence in health care and to continually strive for quality improvements. It is, therefore, imperative that nurses understand the concept of clinical governance and their individual roles and responsibilities within it.

Historically, the government has always been concerned with the organisational management and financial probity of health care, and the NHS has been managed in a variety of ways. The medical profession exerted an enormous influence on the way the NHS was initially set up and managed. However, subsequent health service reforms have attempted to shift the emphasis of power away from the medical profession towards managerial accountability in the 1970s and then towards a market-led framework of financial efficiency in the early 1990s. This evolutionary process has led to the current position whereby all health-care providers have a statutory duty for quality improvement (Scott 2001). The current focus on quality has evolved from recognition that there have been unacceptable variations in performance and practice within the NHS. Examples are inequalities in waiting times for operations, the 'postcode lottery' of treatments available and a lack of national standards for practice (DOH 1998). The government has, therefore, set up a framework for setting, delivering and monitoring standards within the NHS. The aim of the new framework is to provide a service to patients that strives to improve standards of care, improve equity

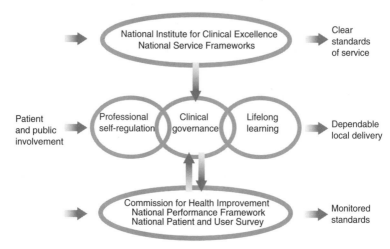

Figure 8.1 Setting, delivering and monitoring standards. (Reproduced from Department of Health 1998 with permission of Her Majesty's Stationery Office.)

of access to services and ensure practice is based on the best evidence available. This framework is set at both local and national levels, and incorporates three main elements (see Fig. 8.1):

- The setting of national quality standards through the development of national service frameworks (NSFs) and the National Institute for Clinical Excellence (NICE).
- Local frameworks of clinical governance to ensure delivery of clinical services that are of high quality and are dependent upon both the continuing professional development of staff (lifelong learning) and professional bodies that ensure that practitioners are fit for practice (professional self-regulation).
- Effective systems for monitoring the quality of services both locally through audit and nationally through the Commission for Health Improvement (CHI).

CLINICAL GOVERNANCE

Clinical governance is at the heart of this framework and has been defined as 'a framework through which NHS organisations are accountable for continuously improving the quality of their services and safeguarding high standards of care by creating an environment in which excellence in clinical care will flourish' (DoH 1998, paragraph 3.2). Under clinical governance, Chief Executives of Trusts are accountable on behalf of NHS Trust Boards for assuring the quality of services. Clinical governance is as much about the way we work as about what we do and how we do it, that is, how we organise our services. Clinical governance has four main components:

- clear lines of responsibility and accountability for the overall quality of clinical care
- a programme of quality improvement activities
- clear policies aimed at managing risks
- procedures for all professional groups to identify and remedy poor performance.

Wherever you work, there will be a named person responsible for the implementation of clinical governance. Each Trust has the scope to implement clinical governance to suit local need and it is your responsibility as a nurse to ensure you understand your role within your organisation's framework. While you are professionally accountable for your practice under the Nursing and Midwifery Council's (NMC's) Code of Professional Conduct (NMC 2002), you are also accountable to your employer and the patient for your practice under the terms of clinical governance.

Activity 8.5
What do you think is your role in relation to adopting clinical governance within your organisation?

You may have mentioned implementing NSF standards locally, how you manage complaints in your clinical area or taking part in clinical audits, such as pressure ulcer audits, as examples of how you have been involved in clinical governance. You may also be involved in projects set up to deal with recommendations following CHI visits or projects involved with delivering the targets set by Health Improvement Programmes (HIMPs) locally. These will all require participation and partnership with other professionals who contribute to the health and social care of the community. They will also necessitate all staff scrutinising their practice to ensure that continual improvements are made and that those with the appropriate skills are delivering the service. The need for innovative solutions for clinical problems may require creative use of resources and may well lead to further blurring of professional boundaries in the future.

The notion of 'closing the loop' is recognised as being imperative in clinical governance. Not only should we be asking 'what are we doing?' and 'how well are we doing it?' but we should also be considering 'how can we do it better?' For example, a complaints procedure should ensure that patients and their families receive timely feedback on any complaint that they might have made, and an audit of complaints can measure whether these have been dealt with in an effective and timely manner. Moreover, 'closing the loop' in this instance would also entail learning from mistakes made and putting new practices into place to avoid recurrence of similar problems in the future. Finally, the question must be asked, 'have we made things better?' Thus, clinical governance is not about setting up a series of committees; it is about everyone being involved in taking responsibility for improving the services delivered to patients to secure the greatest possible improvements in the health of the local population.

Activity 8.6
How has the introduction of clinical governance affected the way care is organised within your clinical area?

Wilson (2002) notes that clinical governance incorporates a number of processes including:

- Clinical audit—this includes local audit and participation in national external audit, e.g. collecting data relating to NSF targets.
- Evidence-based practice in daily use—clinical practice must be evidence based, e.g. the implementation of integrated care pathways (ICPs) or clinical guidelines that are evidence based.
- Clinical effectiveness—a balance needs to be struck between effectiveness, appropriateness and acceptability, e.g. clinical decisions based on NICE guidelines and patient choice.
- Clinical risk management—this pulls together all the elements of clinical governance, and good risk management awareness is crucial at all levels, e.g. prevention and avoidance of untoward incidents and events, changing practices as a result of 'near miss' incidents and unwanted outcomes, and continuing professional development of staff.
- Outcomes of care clearly delineated—clinical audit can only be effective if measurable outcomes are set which can then be audited, e.g. analysis of variance in ICPs is only achievable if clear outcomes are set.
- Good-quality clinical data used to monitor clinical care with early recognition and management of poor practice—data generated must be utilised and acted upon, e.g. pressure ulcer audits can be used following implementation of preventative guidelines to measure whether they are effective in reducing incidence of pressure ulcers.
- Good practice systematically disseminated both within and outside the organisation—the infrastructure must support the dissemination of good practice, e.g. intranet sites and practice development forums.

Health-care organisations must be able to show clear lines of accountability, reporting mechanisms, risk management strategies and ongoing quality enhancement to meet the agenda for clinical governance. Nurses have a crucial role to play at a number of levels in ensuring this agenda is met. They need to use their critical-thinking and decision-making skills to play a part in ensuring care delivered is based on sound evidence, and use their skills of reflection to learn from their experience in order to play their role in introducing and monitoring improvements. Thus, the individual nurse's professional accountability is truly exercised in clinical governance and they have the duty to demonstrate how they are taking this forward in their everyday practice.

SUMMARY

In this chapter, the way nurses organise care has been explored, and some of the advantages and disadvantages of the systems used have been discussed. Emerging roles for nurses have been highlighted in relation to how this can affect the manner in which patient care is managed, especially in relation to interprofessional working. Finally, clinical governance has been outlined and the nurse's role in the processes involved in it have been discussed. It is envisaged that these discussions have highlighted the crucial role that nurses can play in managing care and meeting the health-care agenda for the future.

What is reflective practice?

INTRODUCTION

In the last two decades, there has been an increasing interest in how professionals learn and the ways in which they attempt to describe the epistemology of practice. In particular, tools that may facilitate the integration of theory and practice in the caring professions have been the focus of much debate and speculation. Reflection and reflective practice have been at the heart of many of these discussions, and there is a plethora of literature on the subject in relation to nursing and nurse education. Reflection has generally been considered as a positive process that will enhance nursing practice. The United Kingdom Central Council for Nursing, Midwifery and Health Visiting (UKCC) expects all registered nurses to engage in some form of reflective activity and to keep a personal professional portfolio, which includes reflective accounts of practice (UKCC 1990, 1997b). Additionally, the UKCC Commission for Nursing and Midwifery Education (UKCC 1999, 38) stated that pre-registration students must be able 'to demonstrate critical awareness and reflective practice'. The government has also alluded to the need for professionals to be lifelong learners (Department of Health 1998) and this implies some form of reflective ability is required. In this chapter, therefore, we aim to investigate what reflection and reflective practice entails, and consider its merits and shortcomings. We examine the need for reflection and consider some frameworks that may facilitate the reflective process. The links between reflective practice and critical thinking are examined, and methods to enhance reflection are considered. There is particular emphasis on levels of reflection and how these relate to the skill and experience of the nurse.

INTENDED LEARNING OUTCOMES

By the end of this chapter you will:

1. be able to offer a definition of reflection and discuss the processes involved
2. critically discuss the purported benefits and shortcomings of using reflection as a learning tool
3. differentiate between reflection-on-action and reflection-in-action, and suggest who might use the different approaches
4. describe at least one framework for reflection and outline the critical thinking skills required for its use
5. consider some of the vehicles that might be used to facilitate reflection in practitioners with different levels of experience and expertise.

The terms 'reflection', 'reflective thinking' and 'reflective practice' are used extensively in nursing literature, yet there is no consensus on an exact definition or on what the process entails (Atkins & Murphy 1993, Mackintosh 1998, Teekman 2000). These are discussed in more detail in the forthcoming sections of this chapter but firstly we will explore their historical development.

Reflective practice appears to have its foundations in the cognitive theory of education and Dewey is considered to be one of the first proponents of reflective thinking in the 1930s (Mackintosh 1998). He considered reflective thinking as the process between the recognition and the resolution of a problem, much akin to the positivist research paradigm. However, the notion of reflection did not capture the imagination of nurses until the 1980s and the work of Schön (1983) greatly influenced this interest. It should be noted at this point that much of the work in the area of reflective practice has been developed by general educationalists like Boud et al (1985), Gibbs (1988) and Schön (1983) rather than nurse educationalists, but their theories have been applied to the discipline of nursing.

Activity 9.1

Think about a recent experience you have had in practice where you have cared for a patient with complex problems.
How did you decide what course of action to take in relation to their care?
What theory did you base your decisions upon?
How did you know that the theory was appropriate in this instance?

THE WORK OF SCHÖN

Schön (1983) used the term 'technical rationality' to describe the pure applied science view of professional practice, whereby practitioners apply scientific theory and technique to solve problems in practice. However, he also pointed out that practitioners face complex and multifaceted situations in practice, and that they are often not open to the straightforward and rational application of theory. His main contribution to the discourse on reflective practice was to suggest how professionals cope with the inherent difficulties of the 'swampy lowlands' of everyday practice.

Schön stated that practitioners are taught 'espoused theories' to explain the rationale for practice. However, he contended that, when in practice, 'theories-in-use' govern actual behaviours and that these are generated by practitioners' own theories about practice based on experience and the context of the encounter. These types of theory, he claimed, are very difficult to articulate and may not always be congruent with espoused theories. Furthermore, he coined the term 'reflective practice' to describe the process by which the complex epistemology of practice may be uncovered.

Schön (1983) outlined two types of reflection: reflection-in-action and reflection-on-action. The first of these two is related to thinking actively about what one is doing while one is doing it. The practitioner tries to make sense of an experience by questioning their approach and critiquing it while the action is in progress. This reveals the 'tacit knowledge' (Polyani 1967) being used and helps the practitioner towards a greater understanding of the situation. However, he accepted that knowledge used in practice might be largely intuitive and very difficult for practitioners to verbalise. Furthermore, he noted that very experienced practitioners would be most likely to utilise this type of reflection.

In contrast, reflection-on-action involves a 'cognitive post mortem' (Greenwood 1993), whereby the practitioner looks back on situations, explores the approaches and theories they used, and then analyses their effectiveness. This then facilitates a new understanding of the situation that can be used for reference in future practice encounters.

Schön contended that learning by reflection could be taught and that this was best done by the use of a 'clinical practicum' or a virtual learning experience, where practitioners would not be distracted by the pressures and risks of the real world.

While the influence of Schön's work should not be underestimated, it is not without its critics. Greenwood (1993, 1998), for example, views Schön's work as flawed as it does not take into account the importance of reflection-before-action. She contends that reflection-before-action involves thinking through what one wants to do before it is done, and that this is an important part of professional practice and decision-making. Moreover, Mackintosh (1998) argues that Schön fails to define clearly what is reflective practice and makes no attempt to distinguish between levels of reflection. This is echoed by Burrows (1995), who suggests that many novice nurses would have very limited experiences on which to reflect and that this could influence the development of their reflective skills.

Activity 9.2
What do you consider reflection to be? Do you engage in reflective activities? Do you think there is a difference between reflection and thoughtful practice?

Boud et al (1985, 19) define reflection as 'a generic term for those intellectual and affective activities in which individuals engage to explore their experiences in order to lead to new understandings and appreciations'. They describe how teachers could assist reflection by helping students to return to an experience in order to re-evaluate it and gain new perspectives. They contend that reflection involves deliberate learning, which contrasts with thoughtful musing or anecdotal discussion whereby students may think or talk about an experience but may not gain any new insights.

They propose a model based on Kolb's experiential learning cycle (Kolb & Fry 1975) and outlined three stages of reflection (see Fig. 9.1). The first stage entails returning to the experience and describing it in detail. Boud et al (1985) suggest that the teacher can help the students at this stage by asking them to describe the actual events, rather than what they wished had happened. No judgements should be made at this point, but it is important to help the student or nurse to observe the feelings evoked during the experience.

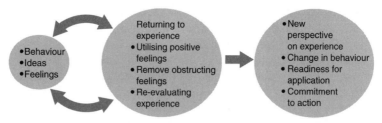

Figure 9.1   Three stages of reflection. (Reproduced from Boud et al 1985 with permission of Kogan Page.)

The second stage involves attending to feelings. Boud et al (1985) suggest that positive feelings can provide the impetus to persist in challenging situations. However, negative feelings can be a barrier to effective learning, and teachers should attempt to help students discharge or transform those feelings in a way that enables them to regain a creative response to the situation.

The third stage is where the experience is re-evaluated. Boud et al (1985) suggest that four aspects need to be considered:

1. Association—the connection of ideas and feelings from the experience being fitted with existing knowledge and attitudes. For example, linking a patient's response to being informed that they have a serious illness to the stages of grieving.

2. Integration—the processing of associations. Relationships are observed and conclusions drawn so that new patterns of ideas and attitudes develop. For example, using knowledge of the patient's social situation to discuss how therapeutic communication skills may help to engender hope in the patient.

3. Validation—new appreciations are tested for internal consistency. Any contradictions lead to reappraisal of the situation. For example, trying to analyse how the plans for engendering hope in the patient previously discussed might work and attempting to identify a range of potential reactions from the patient.

4. Appropriation—new knowledge and perceptions are assimilated into the student's value system. For example, a commitment to trying to help patients cope with distressing news rather than avoiding them in future.

The outcomes of this model may be new perspectives on an experience and a readiness to apply new insights in future. Boud et al (1985) warn that benefits of reflection may be lost, if they are not linked to action, and suggest that the learner should commit to some form of action as a result of their reflections. This may be related to improving a nursing skill or may be a more intellectual activity, such as learning about something that they had identified as a deficit in their knowledge.

Activity 9.3

Think about the last time you reflected upon an experience with a colleague. Were there any strategies they used to help you to make sense of the experience?

Gibbs (1988) relates a framework for structured debriefing to the stages of Kolb's experiential learning cycle (see Fig. 9.2). He notes that, without such structured debriefings, students can jump to premature and often

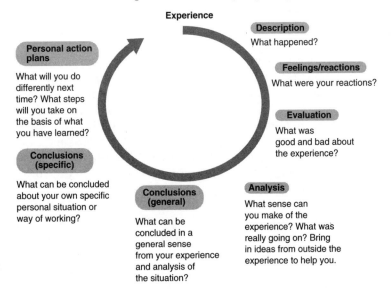

Figure 9.2 Debriefing sequence following experiential learning. (After Gibbs 1988 with permission of OCSLD at Oxford Brookes University.)

erroneous conclusions, or spend so long describing the experience that they do not analyse it.

While these models are clearly educational frameworks firmly grounded in learning from experience, they have been used successfully with nurses. Commitment to action can form the basis of learning contracts with practitioners, clinical supervisors or personal tutors.

An example of a student nurse's reflections using Gibb's (1988) framework is given in Exemplar 1 to illustrate how reflection has enabled a student to develop reflective skills and new insights.

EXEMPLAR 1

Description

I was allocated to work with my mentor, Sarah, in bays 3 and 4 on a late shift. Sarah asked me what I would like to focus on during the shift, and I said I would like to concentrate on two patients and consider their entire care, as I tended to get confused trying to remember everything about all of the patients. She thought this was a good idea and asked me which two patients I would like to focus on. I chose Mr X and Mr Y. We spent some time discussing the care they would require during the afternoon. Sarah said I could observe her doing a dressing on Mr X before supper and then perhaps I could do the dressing under supervision the following day.

Sarah was very busy with the other patients during the shift, and I tried to make myself helpful and not get in the way too much or ask too many questions. At one point, Sarah was talking to a doctor about a patient and I noticed that Mr X's catheter bag was full. I thought I would use my initiative and empty it. I had been taught in school how to do it and Sarah had observed me on the previous shift. I collected the equipment and explained to Mr X what I was doing. Once I had emptied the catheter bag, I took the jug of urine to the sluice and measured it. I then discarded the urine and put the jug in the bedpan washer.

When I went to record the amount of urine on Mr X's fluid balance chart, I noticed that Sarah had finished speaking to the doctor and so I asked her to check that I was charting it correctly. She observed me doing so and then said 'Is the urine in the sluice? We need to keep it for a 24-hour urine collection.' When I told her I had thrown it away, she looked annoyed and said 'I told you he was on a 24-hour urine. We'll have to start another one now.' Then she sent me for my tea break.

Feelings

When I listened to the report I was overwhelmed by all the information and began to feel very anxious. What if I forgot to do something very important? I also felt that I had to show how keen and motivated I was to my mentor. She had worked with me on the previous shift, and had been really supportive and encouraging. She always asked me what I wanted to do and learn even though she was very busy. Sometimes I felt like I was in the way and tried not to follow her everywhere but, as this is my first ward, I did feel quite lost and useless as I realised how little I could do. When I saw that the catheter bag needed emptying, I was excited, as I knew I could safely do that without supervision. I thought Sarah would be pleased at me taking the initiative. When she asked me what I had done with the urine, I was pleased that I could say that I had discarded it, as it showed I had completed the job and cleared up after me. I was mortified when she told me they were supposed to be collecting the urine. I had heard her say 24-hour urine, but I thought that was another term for a fluid balance chart. I felt I had let her down and was very upset that I had made such a stupid mistake. I was upset in my tea break, I felt sick and could not eat or drink anything. I was a bit scared to go back to the ward after my break, but Sarah was OK and discussed the issue and said she had obviously not explained it well enough. Later that shift, she showed me how to do the dressing.

Evaluation

The good thing was that the mistake did not harm the patient. The bad thing was that I looked stupid in front of my mentor and feel even more underconfident than I did before.

Analysis

This situation knocked my confidence, but Sarah said she should have checked I knew what a 24-hour urine collection was. She said I would learn when I needed to ask questions, but how do I know what I do not know? I also realised that the real reason I emptied the catheter bag without discussing it with Sarah first was that I wanted to impress her. I should have had Mr X's well-being foremost in my mind, rather than focusing on trying to impress my mentor.

Conclusions (general)

I should always check with my mentor before I carry out any unsupervised activities.

Conclusions (specific)

While it is important to try to focus my learning and practice my nursing skills, my main priority should be the welfare of my patients. I have learnt today that my eagerness to please and impress others sometimes makes me lose perspective of what is important, that is, it is more important that my patients are safe than that I look good in front of my mentor.

Action plan

In future, even if I think I know what I am doing, I will check it out with someone senior before I do it. I will not try to impress anyone by using my initiative until I have more knowledge and confidence. I will also look up what tests can be done on urine and why they may be done. This should help me to make some more links between my understanding of biology and its use in nursing practice.

It can be seen from the above example that the student has been able to use Gibbs (1988) structured debriefing questions to help her to analyse her experience and try to make sense of it. While the reflective account could be improved in terms of depth of analysis, it certainly demonstrates a degree of self-awareness and a working through of emotions that could block future learning. The student could usefully develop this for written assignments to demonstrate evidence of learning from experience.

Activity 9.4

Think about your own practice and how you use reflection. What usually prompts you to actively engage in reflective activities?

Atkins and Murphy (1994) reviewed the literature on reflection and found that, although there was no consensus on a definition of reflection, there did seem to be a general agreement in the literature that reflection is usually prompted by an awareness of uncomfortable thoughts and feelings. They suggest that three key stages to reflection emerged from the literature. These stages closely follow those suggested by Boud et al (1985) and are delineated as follows:

- awareness of uncomfortable thoughts and feelings
- critical analysis of feelings and knowledge
- new perspectives.

Smith (1998) states that Atkins and Murphy fail to take account of positive thoughts and feelings that may also prompt critical reflection. However, most of the literature they reviewed does focus on learning experiences where nurses have felt that their knowledge, skills or abilities have been lacking. Perhaps a notable exception to this has been Johns' work in trying to reveal the nature of caring (Johns 2001). He describes 11 threads, which form the nature of caring and which have been uncovered during guided reflection with practitioners on both positive and negative experiences. Furthermore, Kim (1999) notes that reflection can be applied to any situation of self-examination and that the term 'critical reflection' should not be interpreted negatively.

Atkins and Murphy (1993) do note that there is an implicit assumption in the literature that certain cognitive and affective skills are necessary to engage in reflection. They suggest that these are:

- self awareness—an ability to appraise honestly how the situation has affected the individual and vice versa
- description—an ability to recollect events and features accurately, and then describe these
- critical analysis—examining a situation, challenging assumptions and exploring alternative courses of thought or action
- synthesis—integration of new and old knowledge to arrive at new perspectives and understanding
- evaluation—judging the worth or value of something.

From an educational point of view, then, it is of paramount importance to facilitate the development of these skills in student nurses, if they do not already possess them. If a nurse does not develop these skills, it could be argued that they will be unable to engage in reflective activities. As a nurse's critical thinking skills develop, they should be able to extend their skills of reflection. This links to the notion of levels of reflection, which are explored in the next section.

LEVELS OF REFLECTION

Nurses practice at differing levels of competence depending on their experience, attitudes and knowledge base (see Ch. 2 for a discussion of Benner's (1984) work in relation to stages of development). It has been suggested by some authors that there are also different levels of reflection depending on the nurse's experience, critical thinking skills and ability to analyse situations.

Goodman (1984) (cited in Burns & Bulman 2000, 178) outlined three levels of reflection that a practitioner may achieve. The first level is limited to technocratic issues of efficiency, effectiveness and accountability, such as examining how a nurse might improve aseptic technique. The second level additionally looks at the implications and consequences of actions. According to Goodman, a nurse reflecting at this level may begin to examine some of their beliefs and explore how these affect their philosophy of care and their relationships with patients and colleagues. The third level of reflection encompasses ethical and political concerns. A nurse may reflect on a difficult ethical dilemma they have faced in a clinical situation and explore possible alternative courses of action and their consequences. However, at this level, they would also question the values on which their organisation is based, for example, examining the tensions between clinical effectiveness, available resources and patient choice. In Exemplar 1, the student demonstrates the ability to reflect at level 1 and is also beginning to move towards level 2 in their attempt to look at how their own needs impact on others.

Kim (1999) suggests a method of critical inquiry that involves three phases: the descriptive phase, the reflective phase, and the critical or emancipatory phase. These phases move the practitioner from a superficial level of reflection through to the final phase, whereby the need for change and plans of how to bring it about are thought through. This model is discussed as a research method, whereby a researcher facilitates the phases with a practitioner and helps to facilitate the changes required. Rolfe et al (2001), however, suggest that it can be used as a model for reflection.

These levels of reflection relate directly to the theory of single- and double-loop learning first introduced by Argyris and Schön (1974). They distinguished between single-loop or instrumental learning, which leaves underlying values and theory unchanged, and double-loop learning, where assumptions are challenged and underlying values changed. Single-loop learning equates generally with descriptive levels of reflection, whereby, for example, a student may learn to improve their communication techniques in certain situations, whereas deeper levels of reflection might challenge the channels of communication that are taken for granted and suggest alternative strategies.

Wong et al (1995) carried out research to assess the level of student reflection from reflective journals and found that students did reflect at different levels. They identified three categories of student ability in relation to reflection: non-reflectors, reflectors and critical reflectors. Non-reflectors were very descriptive and their thinking was concrete, whereas reflectors could identify relationships between prior and new knowledge, and could modify this to new situations. Critical reflectors were able to frame problems in context, and were able to pursue alternative views and possibilities—they drew on prior knowledge, existing information and the literature. This research was focused on students' abilities in relation to written reflective accounts and the findings could be a result of the students' writing abilities rather than their abilities as critical thinkers and reflectors. However, the results are interesting in light of the assumed links between a practitioner's critical thinking skills and their ability to reflect on practice.

CRITIQUES OF REFLECTION

There does seem to be a growing consensus that nurses reflect at differing levels depending upon their degree of experience and their critical-thinking skills. Nevertheless, Cotton (2001) warns that none of the conceptualisations of reflection are politically neutral, and that the current discourses on the nature and levels of reflection tend towards sweeping inclusiveness. This requires that all nurses must reflect and there is an expectation that they will reflect in a manner that conforms to the organisation's wishes. For example, student nurses are expected to submit written reflective accounts that are then 'judged' by academics. Cotton suggests that this process may mean that, instead of freeing nurses to learn from their own unique experience, they may become docile and conforming nurses who think in the way that the institution wants them to. She also draws on Foucault's concept of power-knowledge and contends that power differentials between reflective practitioners and their 'guides', such as clinical supervisors, could mean that the practitioner's views and interpretations are subjugated in favour of their guide's views. Proponents of the need for critical companions or guides, however, might argue against this position on the grounds that a skilful guide will facilitate, rather than direct reflection.

Interestingly, Cotton also notes that as recipients of the reflective practitioners care, patients' views are rarely, if ever, sought. This is notable in the scant research available on the subject and the methods used to determine the impact of practitioner's reflection. Studies seem to be mainly based on self-reports of the influence of reflection on practice (Paget 2001), interviews with nurses to discuss clinical situations (Teekman 2000) and coding of written critical incidents (Smith 1998). While the results of these studies shed some light on how nurses reflect in practice and their perceptions of the impact of this process, there appears to be no evidence of the impact this has on their clinical practice or outcomes for patients. None of the studies mentioned verify the nurses' views of their practice by observation or interviews with patients. The disparity between nurses reflections and their intended actions has also been highlighted in a paper by Page and Meerabeau (2000) who noted that, following reflective sessions held in a coronary care unit, nurses stated that they found the sessions beneficial and that they had a positive influence on their practice. However, the authors noted that, despite the nurses perceiving benefits from the sessions, they did not follow up on areas identified for action in a timely manner. The authors purported that benefits of reflection are lost if they are not consolidated by application and action. They suggested that, while there may be organisational barriers to taking action, further work is required on 'closing the loop' between reflection and action.

Activity 9.5

What factors might influence whether you take action following a reflective exercise? What do you think might enable you to follow up on your intended actions?

REFLEXIVE PRACTICE

Rolfe et al (2001) discuss the development of knowledge as well as skills as a focus for critical reflection. They argue that there is a level of practice beyond Benner's expertise, which is attained by the advanced practitioner reflecting on practice and creating a body of experiential theoretical knowledge. They call this reflexive practice. They claim that experiential theoretical knowledge can convey the rational processes that underpin the intuitive grasp, which Benner proposes cannot be articulated (see Ch. 2 for a full discussion of Benner's (1984) work).

Rolfe et al (2001) have used Kim's model and integrated it with other theorists' work (Borton 1970, Gibbs 1988, Holm & Stephenson 1994, Johns 1998) to develop a framework for reflexive practice (see Table 9.1). The framework enables the practitioner to both learn from reflection-on-action and to focus on how to improve the situation, clearly linking reflection to

Table 9.1   A framework for reflexive practice. (Reproduced from Rolfe et al, *Critical Reflection for Nursing and the Helping Professions: A User's Guide*, 2001, Palgrave, with permission of Palgrave Macmillan)

Descriptive level of reflection	Theory- and knowledge-building level of reflection	Action-oriented (reflexive) level of reflection
What . . .	So what . . .	Now what . . .
. . . is the problem/difficulty/ reason for being stuck/ reason for feeling bad/ reason we don't get on/etc., etc.?	. . . does this tell me/teach me/imply/mean about me/my patient/others/our relationship/my patient's care/the model of care I am using/my attitudes/ my patient's attitudes/ etc, etc.?	. . . do I need to do in order to make things better/stop being stuck/improve my patient's care/resolve the situation/feel better/get on better/etc., etc.?
. . . was my role in the situation?	. . . was going through my mind as I acted?	. . . broader issues need to be considered if this action is to be successful?
. . . was I trying to achieve?	. . . did I base my actions on?	. . . might be the consequences of this action?
. . . actions did I take?	. . . other knowledge can I bring to the situation? • experiential • personal • scientific	
. . . was the response of others?	. . . could/should I have done to make it better?	
. . . were the consequences: • for the patient? • for myself? • for others?	. . . is my new understanding of the situation?	
. . . feelings did it evoke • in the patient? • in myself? • in others?	. . . broader issues arise from the situation?	
. . . was good/bad about the experience?		

action. They propose that the action or change that forms part of reflexive practice in itself becomes the focus of attention for future reflections. Their framework, therefore, facilitates practitioners 'closing the loop'. Exemplar 2 shows a staff nurse's attempt to utilise the reflexive framework of Rolfe et al to analyse an ongoing clinical situation.

Rolfe et al (2001) note that their framework is not intended for novice nurses but for those advanced practitioners endeavouring to articulate the theory embedded in their practice. They suggest the advanced practitioner moves beyond the limitations of intuitive practice and can express methods of practice. This helps to overcome the difficulty of sharing the knowledge embedded in expert practice.

Rolfe et al (2000) also discuss reflection-in-action in some detail and outline the process of 'meta-reflection', which relates to an ability to reflect on the reflection process while it is in progress. This is similar to Clarke et al's (1996) notion of deep reflection, which is a process that allows practitioners to know about what they know and how they acquired that knowledge. They contend that this process enables practitioners to consider the limits of their reflective practice. For example, there may be some aspect of their personal history that makes it difficult for them to confront certain issues and this understanding can enable them to set parameters for their reflective practice. Reflection is *not* about self-analysis without support. Therefore, understanding the limits of reflective practice using deep or meta-reflection can be a means of enhancing professional practice and critical thinking without causing anxiety or feelings of inadequacy within the experienced practitioner.

EXEMPLAR 2
Descriptive level of reflection

The problem

I am an E grade staff nurse working on a busy medical ward. I am a mentor for Jane, a student nurse. Today, while we were on a shift together, she threw away some urine for a patient who was on a 24-hour urine collection.

My role

At the time that she discarded the urine, I was discussing another patient's care with a medical colleague.

What was I trying to achieve?

I was trying to be supportive of the student by discussing her needs, but also not wanting her to feel that I did not trust her to be on her own.

What actions did I take?

I had discussed the care of the patients for whom the student was caring and had told her that Mr X was on a 24-hour urine. I had left her talking to Mr X about his family while I attended to some other patients. When I found out she had thrown away the urine, I sent her on her tea break.

What was the student's response?

She looked very upset when she realised what she had done.

What were the consequences?

The 24-hour urine collection had been commenced 4 hours earlier, so this mistake would delay the results and may delay treatment. The consequences for Jane were that it could knock her confidence in her own abilities.

Feelings it evoked

I felt I had let Jane down, by not supervising her properly and not ensuring that she understood my instructions regarding the 24-hour urine collection. I was angry with myself for showing my annoyance to her.

What was good/bad about the experience?

The delay in the results was not life-threatening for the patient, so that made the situation seem better. However, I felt that this situation had negatively affected my relationship with Jane, who was visibly upset.

Theory and knowledge building reflection

So what does this tell me?

I need to ensure that I clearly set boundaries with students, so that they are aware of what they are able to deal with on their own. I also need to think about my skills in giving feedback to students. I am happy about reinforcing good behaviour, but am still uncomfortable at telling students when they are wrong or in challenging some of their ideas.

What was going through my mind?

I was annoyed that we would have to start the collection again. My annoyance partly stemmed from my fear that this would reflect badly on me.

Sister would be on duty the next day and would expect the collection to be finished. I was also uncomfortable about telling Jane that she had made a mistake, as she obviously felt she had done well and I did not want to be the one to disabuse her of this.

What did I base my actions on?

I thought I would give Jane some time to recover from discovering she had made a mistake. However, I also needed time to think about how to deal with it, so I sent her on her tea break to give me some thinking time.

What other knowledge can I bring to this situation?

I know from the few times that I have worked with Jane that she is very anxious about being on the ward as she has no previous experience in health care; she keeps apologising for her lack of experience. She is also very eager to please and wants to 'fit in'. I know from my teaching and learning course that students can experience a sense of loss of control, confidence and competence in the clinical arena, and that this can make them feel vulnerable and dependent. I am aware that giving negative feedback is something I need to work on, as I find it difficult. I do not like confrontation and do not like upsetting people. However, I also know that taking risks and making mistakes is part of the process of nursing and of the mentorship process. I also recognise that nursing jargon and abbreviations can be confusing. It is not difficult to see how Jane interpreted my abbreviation of '24-hour urine' as needing to record all his urine rather than collect it, as I did not actually use the word collection. In trying to make sense of all the information she was getting, she fitted this in with her knowledge of fluid balance charts and I did not ensure that I checked out her understanding. I also recognise that, as a relatively new E grade, sister's approval is very important to me. I actively seek ways to demonstrate that I merit my promotion.

What could I have done to make it better?

I should have discussed the mistake and its implications for Jane and the patient as soon as I had discovered her error. Sending her off to tea was not a constructive action. It gave her time to dwell on the negative aspects of her performance, without the chance to discuss constructively how she could avoid similar occurrences in the future. I could also have made it into a learning experience by discussing the need for 24-hour urine collections, and this might have helped her to link her biology, pathophysiology and nursing actions together.

What is my new understanding of the situation?

The real problem in this situation was not that the student made a mistake, but that I felt that I had not supervised her adequately and was not able to deal with giving her feedback immediately. I made the situation worse for the student by sending her off the ward. She saw this almost as a punishment for bad behaviour and I had to spend a considerable amount of time with her afterwards to rectify this.

What are the broader issues that arise from this situation?

I need to think about how I can improve my skills in giving feedback to students. I was surprised when I realised that this affects me in other ways. I have difficulty in giving bad news to patients as well. This is an issue that I feel would be appropriate to discuss in my clinical supervision as a means of taking this forward. I also need to get a balance between supporting students on the ward, but also ensuring that the patients remain as the focus for my time. It has also occurred to me that, just as students are going to make mistakes, I will also do so. This is OK as long as I learn from them and that my patients' safety is not put in jeopardy.

Action-oriented (reflexive) reflection

Now what do I need to do in order to stop being stuck?

I resolved the issue when Jane came back from her tea break, by talking it through with her and explaining that I should have dealt with the issue at the time rather than waiting. However, I recognise that, at the time, I needed some space to think. We discussed quite honestly how we both felt we had let each other down, but also discussed the fact that our patient should be the focus of all our actions. I recognise that our discussion was really a damage-limitation exercise and that my lack of skills had inevitably led to unnecessary distress for one of my students. However, in some ways, it has strengthened our relationship and Jane has given me feedback on how I give her feedback! I do feel that I have now been able to confront what the real issue is, and that is my lack of skills and confidence around the area of giving negative feedback. I will bring this to my next clinical supervision meeting and hope that I can discuss some strategies to improve my practice and confront my fears. Additionally, I think that I could ask the sister or link teacher if I could observe them next time they need to give negative feedback to a student or bad news to a patient, as they are both very experienced and I value their support.

What broader issues need to be considered if this action is to be successful?

I need to prepare myself for some of the reactions I might get from students or patients if I give negative feedback. It is not enough to be able to 'deliver the news'. I will also have to be able to manage the consequences. I will need to learn to deal with the possible range of reactions. For example, how might I deal with a student who gets angry or a patient who seems to deny bad news? Next time I have to give negative feedback or bad news I will ensure that I am able to debrief afterwards with a more experienced colleague.

Now what might be the consequences of this action?

I hope that, by discussing this in clinical supervision and by observing more experienced colleagues, I might be able to improve my skills and increase my confidence in this area. I am pleased that I have reached an awareness of an area I need to improve on and feel motivated to do so. I am aware that I might not gain confidence and skills in a short period of time, but feel that this is a manageable challenge, especially as I have the appropriate support mechanisms in place.

While the staff nurse in this exemplar is not at an advanced practitioner level, she has demonstrated new insights into a clinical situation and has already put remedial steps into play to ameliorate the situation with her student. Furthermore, she has identified ways to improve her clinical knowledge and skills further, and has committed to future action and change. She will be able to continue to use the reflexive framework to monitor and reflect upon the identified future actions as they progress.

Activity 9.6
What mechanisms and processes are in place in the organisation in which you work to facilitate reflective practice? Which do you find most beneficial?

USING GUIDES FOR REFLECTION

We have already discussed some models and frameworks that can be used to guide reflective exercises, whether they are verbal reflections or written reflections. However, some theorists propose the use of human 'guides' or critical friends to facilitate the process of reflection. These can be colleagues or facilitators designated by an organisation. The most usual format for facilitated reflection in practice is clinical supervision. It is outside the scope of this chapter to address this in detail but it is discussed elsewhere (see, for example Cutliffe et al 2001, Morton-Cooper & Palmer 2000). It should be noted that clinical supervision is the method favoured by the statutory bodies, who also require practitioners to keep a portfolio (UKCC 1997b). It can be carried out on an individual basis or in groups where supervision can be used to suit the needs of the clinical area.

For pre-registration students, reflective groups and written assignments are the most popular forms of facilitating reflective practice. The skills of reflective writing can be learned and Rolfe et al (2001) assert that reflective writing can enable students to develop their critical-thinking skills by helping them to order their thoughts. It also enables them to make connections between ideas and provide a permanent record, which can be returned to at a later stage for further development. They further suggest different strategies for reflective writing that should suit a variety of writing approaches, such as journal writing, critical incident analyses, writing unsent letters, writing as the other and storytelling. The two exemplars of critical writing offered in this chapter have utilised published frameworks to help structure their progress, and demonstrate how critical-thinking skills and links between ideas can be made through structured reflective writing.

As with any tool, the novice may require more direction in its use than more experienced practitioners, but learning to reflect is not always as easy or straightforward as it may seem initially. It requires sufficient time, thought and often another person to help us when we get 'stuck'. However, perseverance can reap benefits in the pursuit of development of nursing knowledge and skills.

SUMMARY

Reflection has been accepted generally as a vehicle for professional development within the sphere of nursing. It is thought that it develops nurses' critical-thinking skills and their clinical practice. However, it is not without its critics, who maintain that there is limited research to demonstrate any direct link to improved patient outcomes (Burton 2000, Mackintosh 1998) and that it has inherent ethical connotations, if it uncovers poor practice (Cotton 2001, Hannigan 2001).

Nevertheless, in this chapter, we have discussed how reflection can help practitioners to articulate the rationale for their practice, and to seek means of improving their knowledge base and their clinical practice. It can help individuals to examine their values and to challenge some assumptions that are taken for granted about the way in which they work and the organisations that they work for.

We have made links between theories of learning and reflection, and have examined strategies and frameworks devised to promote deeper levels of reflection, as nursing expertise develops. If nurses are to be held accountable for their actions, they must be able to articulate the rationale for their practice. It is hoped that the discussion of reflection in this chapter has helped to elucidate some of the processes that nurses can use to identify the theory embedded in their practice and demonstrate how their practice affects patients. Moreover, it has highlighted the need for further research in this area to examine how reflection impacts on practice and patient outcomes, which also fits with the clinical governance agenda so prominent at the current time.

References

Adams A, Bond S, Hale C. (1998) Nursing organizational practice and its relationship with other features of ward organization and job satisfaction. Journal of Advanced Nursing 27(6): 1212–1222

Alfaro-LeFevre R. (1998) Applying nursing process: a step-by-step guide, 4th edn. Philadelphia: Lippincott

Argyris C, Schön D. (1974) Theory in practice: increasing professional effectiveness. London: Jossey Bass

Arkell S. (1997) Managed care: the benefits and implications for clinical practice. British Journal of Nursing 6(4): 230–233

Atkins S, Murphy K. (1993) Reflection: a review of the literature. Journal of Advanced Nursing 18(8): 1188–1192

Audit Commission. (1991) The virtue of patients: making the most of ward nursing resources. London: HMSO

Auvil-Novak SE. (1997) A middle-range theory of chronotherapeutic intervention for postsurgical pain. Nursing Research 46(2): 66–71

Ballou KA. (1998) A concept analysis of autonomy. Journal of Professional Nursing 14(2): 102–110

Batey M, Lewis F. (1982a) Clarifying autonomy and accountability in nursing service: Part 1. The Journal of Nursing Administration 12(9): 13–18

Batey M, Lewis F. (1982b) Clarifying autonomy and accountability in nursing service: Part 2. The Journal of Nursing Administration 12(10): 10–15

Beauchamp TL, Childress JF. (1994) Principles of biomedical ethics, 4th edn. Oxford: Oxford University Press

Becker C. (1983) A conceptualization of concept. Nursing Papers 15(2): 51–58

Beckstrand J. (1980) A critique of several conceptions of practice theory in nursing. Research in Nursing and Health 3(2): 69–80

Belenky M, Clinchy B, Goldberger N, et al (1986) Women's ways of knowing: the development of self, voice and mind. New York: Basic

Benner P. (1984) From novice to expert: excellence and power in clinical nursing practice. Menlo Park: Addison Wesley

Benner P, ed. (1994) Interpretive phenomenology—embodiment, caring and ethics in health and illness. Thousand Oaks: Sage

Benner P, Wrubel J. (1982) Skilled clinical knowledge: the value of perceptual awareness. Nurse Educator May–June: 11–17

Benner P, Wrubel J. (1989) The primacy of caring, stress and coping in health and illness. Menlo Park: Addison Wesley

Benzein E, Saveman BI. (1998) One step towards the understanding of hope: a concept analysis. International Journal of Nursing Studies 35(6): 322–329

Bergman R. (1981) Accountability—definition and dimensions. International Nursing Review 28(2): 53–59

Binnie A. (2000a) Freedom to practice: patient-centred care. Nursing Times 96(4): 39–40

Binnie A. (2000b) Freedom to practice: establishing continuity. Nursing Times 96(5): 43

Binnie A. (2000c) Freedom to practice: the doctor-nurse relationship. Nursing Times 96(9): 44–46

Borton T. (1970) Reach, touch and teach. London: McGraw–Hill

Boud D, Keogh R, Walker D. (1985) Promoting reflection in learning: a model. In: Boud D, Keogh R, Walker D, eds. Reflection: turning experience into learning. London: Kogan Page: 18–40

Boychuk Duschscher J. (1999) Catching the wave: understanding the concept of critical thinking. Journal of Advanced Nursing 29(3): 577–583

Burns N, Groves SK. (2001) The practice of nursing research, conduct, critique and utilization, 4th edn. Philadelphia: Saunders

Burns S, Bulman C, eds. (2000) Reflective practice in nursing, 2nd edn. Oxford: Blackwell Science

Burrows D. (1995) The nurse teacher's role in the promotion of reflective practice. Nurse Education Today 15(5): 346–350

Burton A. (2000) Reflection: nursing's practice and education panacea? Journal of Advanced Nursing 31(5): 1009–1017

Carper BA. (1978) Fundamental patterns of knowing in nursing. Advances in Nursing Science 1(1): 13–23

Castledine G. (1986) A stress adaptation model. In: Kershaw B, Salvage J, eds. Models for nursing. Chichester: Wiley

Chambers (1995) Chambers combined dictionary thesaurus. Edinburgh: Chambers Harrap

Chinn PL, Jacobs MK. (1987) Theory and nursing: a systematic approach, 2nd edn. St Louis: Mosby

Chinn PL, Kramer MK. (1991) Theory and nursing—a systematic approach, 3rd edn. St Louis: Mosby

Chinn PL, Kramer MK. (1995) Theory and nursing—a systematic approach, 4th edn. St Louis: Mosby

Chinn PL, Kramer MK. (1999) Theory and nursing, 5th edn. St Louis: Mosby

Cioffi J. (2002) What are clinical judgements? In: Thompson C, Dowding D, eds. Clinical decision making and judgement in nursing. Edinburgh: Churchill Livingstone: 47–65

Clark J, Lang N. (1992) Nursing's next advance: an international classification for nursing practice. International Nursing Review 38(4): 109–112

Clarke B, James C, Kelly J. (1996) Reflective practice: reviewing the issues and refocusing the debate. International Journal of Nursing Studies 33(2): 171–180

Coady E. (2002) Chronic heart failure 3. Initiatives in coronary care services. Nursing Times 98(30): 41–44

Coombs M, Dillon A. (2002) Crossing boundaries, re-defining care: the role of the critical care outreach team. Journal of Clinical Nursing 11(3): 387–393

Cotton A. (2001) Private thoughts in public spheres: issues in reflection and reflective practices in nursing. Journal of Advanced Nursing 36(4): 512–519

Cutcliffe J, Butterworth T, Proctor B, eds. (2001) Clinical supervision. London: Routledge

Cutliffe JR, Herth K. (2002a) The concept of hope in nursing 1: its origins, background and nature. British Journal of Nursing 11(12): 832–840

Cutliffe JR, Herth K. (2002b) The concept of hope in nursing 2: hope and mental health nursing. British Journal of Nursing 11(13): 885–893

Cutliffe JR, Herth K. (2002c) The concept of hope in nursing 3: hope and palliative care nursing. British Journal of Nursing 11(14): 977–983

Daly W. (1998) Critical thinking as an outcome of nursing education. What is it? Why is it important to nursing practice? Journal of Advanced Nursing 28(2): 323–331

Davies C. (1996) A new vision of professionalism. Nursing Times 92(46): 54–56

Dealey C. (1999) The care of wounds—a guide for nurses, 2nd edn. London: Blackwell

de la Cuesta C. (1983) The nursing process: from development to implementation. Journal of Advanced Nursing 8(5): 365–371

de Luc K. (2000) Care pathways: an evaluation of their effectiveness. Journal of Advanced Nursing 32(2): 485–496

Department of Health (1977) DoH circular: The extended role of the nurse. London: Department of Health

Department of Health (1991) The patient's charter. London: HMSO

Department of Health (1995) The nursing and therapy professions' contribution to health services research and development. London: Department of Health

Department of Health (1997) The new NHS: modern, dependable. London: The Stationery Office

Department of Health (1998) A first class service: quality in the new NHS. London: The Stationery Office

Department of Health (2000) National service framework for coronary heart disease. London: Department of Health

Department of Health (2001a) The essence of care: patient-focused benchmarking for health care practitioners. London: Department of Health

Department of Health (2001b) Your guide to the NHS. London: The Stationery Office

Dewey J. (1934) Art as experience. New York: Pedigree

Dickoff J, James P. (1968) A theory of theories: a position paper. Nursing Research 17(3): 197–203

Dickoff J, James P, Wiedenbach E. (1968) Theory in a practice discipline. Part 1. Practice oriented theory. Nursing Research 17(5): 415–435

Dooley F. (1999) The named nurse in practice. Nursing Standard 13(34): 33–38

Drevdahl D. (1999) Sailing beyond: nursing theory and the person. Journal of Advanced Nursing 21(4): 1–13

Dunn L. (1997) A literature review of advanced clinical nursing practice in the United States of America. Journal of Advanced Nursing 25(4): 814–819

Eakes GG, Burke ML, Hainsworth MA. (1998) Middle-range theory of chronic sorrow. Image Journal of Nursing Scholarship 30(2): 179–184

Edwards SD. (1998) The art of nursing. Nursing Ethics 5(5): 393–400

Edwards S. (2001) Philosophy of nursing: an introduction. Basingstoke: Palgrave

Engstrom JL. (1984) Problems in the development, use and testing of nursing theory. Journal of Nursing Education 23(6): 245–251

Ersser S, Tutton E, eds. (1991) Primary nursing in perspective. London: Scutari Press

Fawcett J. (1984) The metaparadigm of nursing: present status and future refinements. Image Journal of Nursing Scholarship 16(3): 84–87

Fawcett J. (1989) Analysis and evaluation of conceptual models of nursing, 2nd edn. Philadelphia: Davis

Fawcett J. (1995) Analysis and evaluation of conceptual models of nursing, 3rd edn. Philadelphia: Davis

Fawcett J. (2000) Analysis and evaluation of contemporary nursing knowledge, nursing models and theories. Philadelphia: Davis

Fawcett J, Downs FS. (1992) The relationship of theory and research, 2nd edn. Philadelphia: Davis

Fawcett J, Watson J, Neuman B et al. (2001) On nursing theories and evidence. Journal of Nursing Scholarship 33(2): 115–119

Fealy GM. (1997) The theory-practice relationship in nursing: an exploration of contemporary discourse. Journal of Advanced Nursing 25(5): 1061–1069

Finlay T. (2000) The scope of professional practice: a literature review to determine the document's impact on nurses' role. NT Research 5(2): 115–125

Gibbs G. (1988) Learning by doing: a guide to teaching and learning methods. Oxford: Further Education Unit, Oxford Polytechnic

Gill P, Ryan J, Morgan O. et al. (2000) Team nursing and ITU—a good combination? Intensive and Critical Care Nursing 16(4): 243–255

Gilligan C (1982) In a different voice. Cambridge MA: Harvard University Press

Glaser BG, Strauss AL. (1967) The discovery of grounded theory; strategies for qualitative research. Chicago: Adline

Good M. (1998) A middle range theory of acute pain management; use in research. Nursing Outlook 46(3): 120–124

Good M, Moore SM. (1996) Clinical practice guidelines as a new source of middle range theory: focus on acute pain. Nursing Outlook 44(2): 74–79

Gortner SR. (1990) Nursing values and science: toward a science philosophy. Image Journal of Nursing Scholarship 22(2): 101–105

Greenwood J. (1993) Reflective practice: a critique of the work of Argyris and Schön. Journal of Advanced Nursing 18(8): 1183–1187

Greenwood J. (1998) The role of reflection in single and double loop learning. Journal of Advanced Nursing 27(5):1048–1053

Haase JE, Britt T, Coward DC, et al. (1992) Simultaneous concept analysis of spiritual perspective hope, acceptance and self-transcendence. Image Journal of Nursing Scholarship 24(2): 141–147

Hampton D. (1994) Expertise: the true essence of nursing art. Advances in Nursing Science 17(1): 15–24

Hamric AB, Spross JA, Hanson CH, eds. (1996) Advanced nursing practice: an integrative approach. Philadelphia: Saunders

Hams SP. (1997) Concept analysis of trust: a coronary care perspective. Intensive and Critical Care 13(6): 351–356

Hannigan B. (2001) A discussion of the strengths and weaknesses of 'reflection' in nursing practice and education. Journal of Clinical Nursing 10(2): 278–283

Haralambos M, Holborn M. (2000) Sociology themes and perspectives, 5th edn. London: Collins

Hardwick S. (1998) Clarification of nursing diagnosis from a British perspective. Assignment – ongoing work of health care students 4(2): 3–9

Heath H. (1998) Reflections and patterns of knowing in nursing. Journal of Advanced Nursing 27(5): 1054–1059

Heidegger M. (1982) The basic problems of phenomenology. (Translated by Hofstader A.) Bloomington: Indiana University Press

Henderson V. (1966) The nature of nursing: a definition and its implications for practice, education and research. London: Collier Macmillan

Herth K. (1990) Fostering hope in terminally-ill people. Journal of Advanced Nursing 15(11): 1250–1259

Hicks C. (1998) The randomised controlled trial: a critique. Nurse Researcher 6(1): 19–32

Hilton P, Goddard M. (1996) Taken to task. Nursing Times 92(16): 44–45

Hogston R.(1997) Nursing diagnosis and classification systems: a position paper. Journal of Advanced Nursing 26(3): 496–500

Holm D, Stephenson S. (1994) Reflection—a student's perspective. In: Palmer A, Burns S, Bulman C. eds. Reflective practice in nursing. Oxford : Blackwell Scientific: 53–62

Hupcey JE, Penrod J, Morse JM et al. (2001) An exploration and advancement of the concept of trust. Journal of Advanced Nursing 36(2): 282–293

Illich I. (1977) Disabling professions. London: Marion Boyars

Jacox A. (1974) Theory construction in nursing: an overview. Nursing Research 23(1): 4–13

Jemmott LS, Jemmott JB III. (1991) Applying the theory of reasoned action to Aids risk behaviour: condom use among black women. Nursing Research 40(4): 228–234

Johns C. (1998) Opening the doors of perception. In: Johns C, Freshwater, D. eds. Transforming nursing through reflective practice. Oxford: Blackwell Science: 1–20

Johns C. (2001) Reflective practice: revealing the [he]art of caring. International Journal of Nursing Practice 7(4): 237–245

Johns JL. (1996) A concept analysis of trust. Journal of Advanced Nursing 24(1): 76–83

Johnson B, Webber P. (2001) Theory and reasoning in nursing. Philadelphia: Lippincott

Johnson JL. (1994) A dialectical examination of nursing art. Advances in Nursing Science 17(1): 1–14

Johnson JL. (1996) Dialectical analysis concerning the rational aspect of the art of nursing. Image Journal of Nursing Scholarship 28(2): 169–175

Johnson S, Smith J. (2000) Factors influencing the success of ICP projects. Professional Nurse 15(12): 776–779

Johnson S , Dracass M, Vartan J. et al. (2000) Setting standards using integrated care pathways. Professional Nurse 15(10): 640–643

Kataoka-Yahiro M, Saylor C. (1994) A critical thinking model for nursing judgement. Journal of Nursing Education 33(8): 351–356

Kenny G. (2002) The importance of nursing values in interprofessional collaboration. British Journal of Nursing 11(1): 65–68

Kidd P, Morrison EF. (1988) The progression of knowledge in nursing: a search for meaning. Image Journal of Nursing Scholarship 20(4): 222–224

Kim H. (1999) Critical reflective inquiry for knowledge development in nursing practice. Journal of Advanced Nursing 29(5): 1205–1212

King I. (1971) Towards a theory for nursing: general concepts of human behaviour. New York: Wiley

King I. (1981) A theory for nursing: systems, concepts, process. New York: Wiley

King I. (1988) Concepts: essential elements of theories. Nursing Science Quarterly 1(1): 22–25

Klages M. (1997) Postmodernism http://www.colorado.edu.English/ENGL2012Klages/pomo.html (accessed 10.05.2002)

Kolb D, Fry R. (1975) Towards an applied theory of experiential learning. In Cooper CL. ed. Theories of group processes. London: Wiley: 33–57

Kramer MK. (1993) Concept clarification and critical thinking: integrated processes. Journal of Nursing Education 32(9): 406–414

Kuhn T. (1970) The structure of scientific revolutions, 2nd edn. Chicago: University of Chicago Press

Kylmä J, Vehviläinen-Julkunen K. (1997) Hope in nursing research: a meta-analysis of the ontological and epistemological foundations of research on hope. Journal of Advanced Nursing 25(2): 364–369

Landers MG. (2000) The theory–practice gap in nursing: the role of the nurse teacher. Journal of Advanced Nursing 32(6): 1550–1556

Lawson N. (1996) Irrelevant academic qualifications are an insult to nurses—and useless to their patients. The Observer, 26th December 1996

Laxade S, Hale C. (1995a) Managed care 1: an opportunity for nursing. British Journal of Nursing 4(5): 290–294

Laxade S, Hale C.(1995b) Managed care 2: an opportunity for nursing. British Journal of Nursing 4(6): 345–350

Leaper DJ. (1992) Eusol. British Medical Journal 304(6832): 930–931

Leddy S, Pepper M. (1998) Conceptual bases of professional nursing, 4th edn. Philadelphia: Lippincott

Leininger M. (1985) Nature, rationale and importance of qualitative research methods in nursing. In: Leininger M, ed. Qualitative research methods in nursing. Orlando: Grune & Stratton: 1–26

Lenz ER, Suppe F, Gift A et al. (1995) Collaborative development of middle-range nursing theories: towards a theory of unpleasant symptoms. Advances in Nursing Science 17(3): 1–13

Leonard VW. (1989) A Heideggarian phenomenological perspective on the concept of person. Advances in Nursing Science 11(4): 40–55

Levine ME. (1995) The rhetoric of nursing theory. Image Journal of Nursing Scholarship 27(1): 11–14

Liehr P, Smith, MJ. (1999) Middle-range theory: spinning research and practice to guide knowledge for the new millennium. Advances in Nursing Science 21(4): 81–91

Lindsay B. (1990) The gap between theory and practice. Nursing Standard 5(4): 34–35

Lo-Biondo-Wood G, Haber J. (1998) Nursing research, methods, critical appraisal and utilization, 4th edn. St Louis: Mosby

Lowe C. (1998) Care pathways: have they a place in 'the new National Health Service'? Journal of Nursing Management 6(5): 303–306

Lutzen K, Tishelman C. (1996) Nursing diagnosis: a critical analysis of underlying assumptions. International Journal of Nursing Studies 33(2): 190–200

MacDonald C. (2002) Nurse autonomy as relational. Nursing Ethics 9(2): 194–201

Macdonald K. (1997) The sociology of the professions. London: Sage

Mackintosh C. (1998) Reflection: a flawed strategy for the nursing profession. Nurse Education Today 18(7): 553–557

Manthey M. (1992) The practice of primary nursing. London: The King's Fund Centre

Maquis Bishop S. (1989) Theory development process. In: Marriner-Tomey A, ed. Nursing theorists and their work, 2nd edn. St Louis: Mosby: 40–50

Marriner-Tomey A. (1998) Nursing theorists and their work, 4th edn. St Louis: Mosby

Maslow AH. (1954) Motivation and personality. New York: Harper and Row

Masterson A. (2002) Cross-boundary working: a macropolitical analysis of the impact on professional roles. Journal of Clinical Nursing 11(3): 331–339

McGee P, Castledine G, Brown R. (1996) A survey of specialist and advanced nursing practice in England. British Journal of Nursing 5(11): 682–686

McKay RP. (1969) Theories, models and systems for nursing. Nursing Research 18(5): 393–399

McKenna H. (1997) Nursing theories and models. London: Routledge

McNeil P, Townley C, eds. (1986) Fundamentals of sociology. Cheltenham: Stanley Thornes

Meerabeau L. (1997) 'Why are our grant applications continually rejected?' Nurse Researcher 5(1): 5–14

Meize-Grochowski R. (1984) An analysis of the concept of trust. Journal of Advanced Nursing 9(6): 563–572

Meleis AI. (1985) International nursing for knowledge development. Nursing Outlook 33(3): 144–147

Meleis AI. (1991) Theoretical nursing: development and progress, 2nd edn. Philadelphia: Lippincott

Meleis AI. (1997) Theoretical nursing:development and progress, 3rd edn. Philadelphia: Lippincott

Merleau-Ponty M. (1962) The phenomenology of perception. (Translated by Smith C.) London: Routledge

Merton R K. (1968) Social theory and social structure. New York: Free Press

Moody LE. (1990) Advancing nursing science through research, Vol. 1. Newbury Park: Sage

Morton-Cooper A, Palmer A, eds. (2000) Mentoring, preceptorship and clinical supervision, 2nd edn. Oxford: Blackwell Science

Morse JM. (1995) Exploring the theoretical basis of nursing using advanced techniques of concept analysis. Advances in Nursing Science 17(3): 31–46

Morse JM, Doberneck B. (1995) Delineating the concept of hope. Image Journal of Nursing Scholarship 27(4): 277–285

Morse JM, Mitcham C, Hupcey JE et al. (1996) Criteria for concept evaluation. Journal of Advanced Nursing 24(2): 385–390

Munhall P (1993) 'Unknowing': towards another pattern of knowing in nursing. Nursing Outlook 41(3): 125–128

Nelms TP, Lane EB. (1999) Women's ways of knowing in nursing and critical thinking. Journal of Professional Nursing 15(3): 179–186

Neuman B. (1995) The Neuman's systems model, 3rd edn. Norwalk: Appleton Lange

Newman MA. (1994) Health as expanding consciousness, 2nd edn. New York: National League for Nursing

Norris A, Briggs J. (1999) Care pathways and the information for health strategy. Health Informatics Journal 5(4): 209–212

Nursing and Midwifery Council (2002) Code of Professional Conduct. London: Nursing and Midwifery Council

O'Connell B.(1998) The clinical application of the nursing process in selected acute care settings: a professional mirage. Australian Journal of Advanced Nursing 15(4): 22–32

Olson J, Hanchett E. (1997) Nurse-expressed empathy, patient outcomes, and development of a middle-range theory. Image Journal of Nursing Scholarship 29(1): 71–76

Orem DE. (1971) Nursing: concepts of practice. New York: McGraw-Hill

Orem DE. (1995) Nursing: concepts of practice, 5th edn. St Louis: Mosby

Orem DE. (2001) Nursing: concepts of practice, 6th edn. St Louis: Mosby

Orlando IJ. (1961) The dynamic nurse-patient relationship: function, process and principles. New York: Putnam (Reprinted 1990. New York: National League for Nursing)

Osborn e R. (1992) Philosophy for beginners. New York: Writer and Readers

Page S, Meerabeau L.(2000) Achieving change through reflective practice : closing the loop. Nurse Education Today 20(5): 365–372

Paget T. (2001) Reflective practice and clinical outcomes: practitioners' views on how reflective practice has influenced their clinical practice. Journal of Clinical Nursing 10(2): 204–214

Paley J. (1996) How not to clarify concepts in nursing. Journal of Advanced Nursing 24(3): 572–578

Parahoo K. (1997) Nursing research, principles, process and issues. London: Macmillan

Parse RR. (1981) Man-living-health: a theory for nursing. New York: Wiley

Parse RR. (1987) Nursing science: major paradigms, theories and critiques. Philadelphia: Saunders

Parse RR. (1998) The human becoming school of thought: a perspective for nurses and other health professionals. Thousand Oaks: Sage

Pattison S. (2001) Are nursing codes of practice ethical? Nursing Ethics 8(1): 5–18

Pearson A, ed. (1988) Primary nursing: nursing in the Burford and Oxford nursing development units. London: Chapman and Hall

Penrod J, Morse JM. (1997) Strategies for assessing and fostering hope: the hope assessment guide. Oncology Nursing Forum 24(6): 1055–1063

Peplau H. (1952) Interpersonal relations in nursing. New York: Putnam

Peplau H. (1988) The art and science of nursing: similarities, differences and relations. Nursing Science Quarterly 1(1): 8–15

Pierson W. (1999) Considering the nature of intersubjectivity within professional nursing. Journal of Advanced Nursing 30(2): 294–302

Polanyi M. (1958) Personal knowledge. London: Routledge Kegan Paul

Polyani M. (1967) The tacit dimension. London: Routledge Kegan Paul

Pontin D. (1999) Primary nursing: a mode of care or a philosophy of nursing? Journal of Advanced Nursing 29(3): 584–591

Porter S. (1992) The poverty of professionalisation: a critical analysis of strategies for the occupational advancement of nursing. Journal of Advanced Nursing 17(6): 720–726

Pryjmachuk S. (1996) A nursing perspective on the interrelationships between theory, research and practice. Journal of Advanced Nursing 23(4): 679–684

Quine WVO. (1980) From a logical point of view. London: Harvard University Press

Quine WVO, Ullian JS. (1978) The web of belief. New York: Random House

Reed PG. (1991) Toward a nursing theory of self-transcendence: deductive reformulation using developmental theories. Advances in Nursing Science 13(4): 64–77

Reed PG. (1995) A treatise on nursing knowledge development for the 21st century: beyond postmodernism. Advances in Nursing Science 17(3): 70–84

Reynolds J. (2001) The internet encyclopedia of philosophy—Maurice Merleau-Ponty (1908–1961). http://www.utm.edu/research/iep/merleau.htm (accessed 23.05.2002)

Reynolds PD. (1971) Primer in theory construction. Indianapolis: Bobbs-Merrill

Rodgers BL. (2000) Concept analysis: an evolutionary view. In: Rodgers BL, Knafl KA, eds. Concept development in nursing: foundations, techniques and applications, 2nd edn. Philadelphia: Saunders: 77–102

Rogers M. (1970) An introduction to the theoretical basis of nursing. Philadelphia: Davis

Rolfe G. (1997) Beyond expertise: theory, practice and the reflexive practitioner. Journal of Clinical Nursing 6(2): 93–97

Rolfe G. (1998) The theory-practice gap in nursing: from research-based practice to practitioner-based research. Journal of Advanced Nursing 28(3): 672–679

Rolfe G. (2000) Research, truth, authority—postmodern perspectives on nursing. Basingstoke: Macmillan

Rolfe G, Freshwater D, Jasper M. (2001) Critical reflection for nursing and the helping professions: a user's guide. Houndmills: Palgrave

Roper N, Logan W, Tierney A. (1980) The elements of nursing. Edinburgh: Churchill Livingstone

Roper N, Logan W, Tierney A. (1996) The elements of nursing, 4th edn. Edinburgh: Churchill Livingstone

Roy C. (1971) Adaptation: a basis for nursing practice. Nursing Outlook 18(3): 42–45

Roy C. (1980) The Roy adaptation model. In: Riehl JP and Roy C, eds. Conceptual models for nursing practice, 2nd edn. New York: Appelton–Century–Crofts: 179–188

Roy C. (1984) Introduction to nursing: an adaptation model, 2nd edn. Englewood Cliffs: Prentice-Hall

Roy C, Andrews HA. (1999) The Roy adaptation model, 2nd edn. Stamford: Appleton & Lange

Rustøen T, Hanestad BR. (1998) Nursing intervention to increase hope in cancer patients. Journal of Clinical Nursing 7(1): 19–27

Scheffler I. (1965) Conditions of knowledge: an introduction to epistemology and education. Glenview: Scott Foresman

Scholes J, Vaughan B. (2002) Cross-boundary working: implications for the multiprofessional team. Journal of Clinical Nursing 11(3): 399–408

Schön D. (1983) The reflective practitioner: how professionals think in action. New York: Basic Books

Schriefer J, Botter M. (2001) Nurse case management skills required for care management. Outcomes Management for Nursing Practice 5(2): 48–51

Schröck RA. (1990) Conscience and courage—a critical examination of professional conduct. Nurse Education Today 10: 3–9

Schultz PR, Meleis AI. (1988) Nursing epistemology: traditions, insights, questions. Image Journal of Nursing Scholarship 20(4): 217–221

Scott I. (2001) Clinical governance: a framework and models for practice. In: Bishop V, Scott I, eds. Challenges in clinical practice: professional developments in nursing. Houndmills: Palgrave: 37–58

Sigsworth J. (1995) Feminist research: its relevance to nursing. Journal of Advanced Nursing 22(5): 896–899

Silva MC. (1977) Philosophy, science, theory: interrelationships and implications for nursing research 9(3): 59–63

Silva MC, Sorrell JM, Sorrell CD. (1995) From Carper's patterns of knowing to ways of being: an ontological philosophical shift in nursing. Advances in Nursing Science 18(1): 1–13

Smith A. (1998) Learning about reflection. Journal of Advanced Nursing 28(4): 891–898

Solomon RC. (1985) From rationalism to existentialism—the existentialists and their nineteenth-century backgrounds, 2nd edn. Maryland: Littlefield Adams

Stephenson C. (1991) The concept of hope revisited for nursing. Journal of Advanced Nursing 16(12): 1456–1461

Steven A. (1999) Named nursing: in whose best interest? Journal of Advanced Nursing 29(2): 341–347

Stevens-Barnum BJ. (1994) Nursing theory: analysis, application, evaluation, 4th edn. Philadelphia: Lippincott

Stevens-Barnum BJ. (1998) Nursing theory: analysis, application, evaluation, 5th edn. Philadelphia: Lippincott

Taylor BJ. (1993) Phenomenology: one way to understand nursing practice. International Journal of Nursing Studies 30(2): 171–179

Taylor BJ. (1994) Being human—ordinariness in nursing. Melbourne: Churchill Livingstone

Taylor C. (1997) Problem solving in clinical nursing practice. Journal of Advanced Nursing 26(2): 329–336

Taylor C. (2000) Clinical problem solving in nursing: insights from the literature. Journal of Advanced Nursing 31(4): 842–849

Taylor P, Richardson J, Yeo A et al. (1995) Sociology in focus. Lancashire: Causeway Press

Teekman B. (2000) Exploring reflective thinking in nursing practice. Journal of Advanced Nursing 31(5): 1125–1135

Thompson C. (1999) A conceptual treadmill: the need for 'middle ground' in clinical decision making theory in nursing. Journal of Advanced Nursing 30(5): 1222–1229

Thompson C, Dowding D.(2002) Decision making and judgement in nursing—an introduction. In: Thompson C , Dowding D, eds. Clinical decision making and judgement in nursing. Edinburgh: Churchill Livingstone: 1–20

Thorne S, Canam C, Dahinten S et al. (1998) Nursing's metaparadigm concepts: disempacting the debates. Journal of Advanced Nursing 27(6): 1257–1268

Timpson J. (1996) Nursing theory: everything the artist spits is art? Journal of Advanced Nursing 23(5): 1030–1036

Tschudin V, Hunt G. (1998) Editorial. Nursing Ethics 5: 383–384

United Kingdom Central Council for Nurses, Midwives and Health Visitors (1989) Nurses, Midwives and Health Visitors Amendment Approval Order (Rule 18A(2)). London: UKCC

United Kingdom Central Council for Nurses, Midwives and Health Visitors (1990) The report of the post registration education and practice project. London: UKCC

United Kingdom Central Council for Nurses, Midwives and Health Visitors (1992a) Code of professional conduct for the nurse, midwife and health visitor. London: UKCC

United Kingdom Central Council for Nurses, Midwives and Health Visitors (1992b) The scope of professional practice. London: UKCC

United Kingdom Central Council for Nurses, Midwives and Health Visitors (1997a) PREP— the nature of advanced practice. CC/97/06. London: UKCC

United Kingdom Central Council for Nurses, Midwives and Health Visitors (1997b) PREP and you. London: UKCC

United Kingdom Central Council for Nurses, Midwives and Health Visitors (1999) Fitness for practice. The UKCC Commission for Nursing and Midwifery Education (Chair: Sir Leonard Peach). London: UKCC

Uys LR. (1987) Foundational studies in nursing. Journal of Advanced Nursing 12(3): 275–280
van Hooft S. (1998) The art of nursing: aesthetics or praxis? A response to Steven Edwards, Louise de Raeve and Per Nortvedt. Nursing Ethics 5: 545–550
Varcoe C. (1996) Disparagement of the nursing process: the new dogma? Journal of Advanced Nursing 23(1): 120–125
von Bertalanffy L. (1956) General system theory. Yearbook of the Society for the Advancement of General System Theory 1(1): 1–10
von Bertalanffy L. (1968) General system theory. New York: Braziller
Wade G. (1999) Professional nurse autonomy: concept analysis and application to nursing education. Journal of Advanced Nursing 30(2): 310–318
Wainwright P. (2000) Towards an aesthetics of nursing. Journal of Advanced Nursing 32(3): 750–756
Walker LO. (1992) Towards a clearer understanding of the concept of nursing theory. In: Nicholl LH, ed. Perspectives on nursing theory, 2nd edn. London: Lippincott: 29–39
Walker LO, Avant KC. (1983) Strategies for theory construction in nursing. Norwalk: Appleton & Lange
Walker LO, Avant KC. (1995) Strategies for theory construction in nursing, 3rd edn. Norwalk: Appleton & Lange
Walsh M. (1997) Will critical pathways replace the nursing process? Nursing Standard 11(52): 39–42
Walsh M. (2000) Nursing frontiers: accountability and the boundaries of care. Oxford: Butterworth-Heinemann
Waters K, Easton N. (1999) Individualized care: is it possible to plan and carry out? Journal of Advanced Nursing 29(1): 79–87
Watson J. (1981) Nursing's scientific quest. Nursing Outlook 29(7): 413–416
Watson J. (1988) Nursing: human science and human care. New York: National League for Nursing
Westman RS. (2002) 'Nicolaus Copernicus' Microsoft@Encarta ®Online Encyclopaedia 2002 http://encarta.msn.com © 1997–2002 Microsoft Corporation, All rights reserved
White J. (1995) Patterns of knowing: review, critique and update. Advances in Nursing Science 17(4): 73–86
Whittemore R. (1999a) Natural science and nursing science: where do the horizons fuse? Journal of Advanced Nursing 30(5): 1027–1033
Whittemore, R. (1999b) To know is to act knowledge (Analects 2,17). Journal of Nursing Scholarship 31(4): 365–366
Wilkinson J. (1997) Developing a concept analysis of autonomy in nursing practice. British Journal of Nursing 6(12): 703–707
Wilson J. (1963) Thinking with concepts. New York: Cambridge University Press
Wilson J. (2002) Clinical governance: the legal perspective. In: Tingle J, Cribb A, eds. Nursing law and ethics, 2nd edn. Oxford: Blackwell Science: 224–239
Wilson-Barnett J, Barriball L, Reynolds H et al. (2000) Recognising advancing nursing practice: evidence from two observational studies. International Journal of Nursing Studies 37(5): 389–400
Wong F, Kember D, Chung L et al. (1995) Assessing the level of student reflection from reflective journals. Journal of Advanced Nursing 22(1): 48–57

Index

Page numbers in **bold** refer to figures, and those in *italic* to tables.